Diet Fads, Careers & Controversies in Nutrition Journalism

Diet Fads, Careers & Controversies in Nutrition Journalism

✦

How to Organize Term Papers, News, or Debates

Anne Hart

ASJA Press
New York Lincoln Shanghai

Diet Fads, Careers & Controversies in Nutrition Journalism
How to Organize Term Papers, News, or Debates

Copyright © 2005 by Anne Hart

ASJA Press
an imprint of iUniverse, Inc.

iUniverse books may be ordered through booksellers or by contacting:

iUniverse
2021 Pine Lake Road, Suite 100
Lincoln, NE 68512
www.iuniverse.com
1-800-Authors (1-800-288-4677)

ISBN-13: 978-0-595-37823-4

ISBN-10: 0-595-37823-4

Printed in the United States of America

Contents

1

Adolescent and Childhood Obesity Issues

Do you need to write a school term paper on nutrition? Are you interested in how to start or train for a career, get a job, or open businesses writing or speaking about nutrition, health, or consumer economics communications? Or do you need to explain to adolescents, college students, or children about the epidemic of diabetes and obesity?

How do you start a career, get a job, or open businesses writing or speaking about scientifically-substantiated plant extracts? Can you bridge the gap between science and the consumer with understandable explanations? Diabetes is expected to surpass cancer and heart disease as America's leading killer by 2010.

How are you going to write or talk about this epidemic for the average consumer of news? Are you going to tell people how to control their blood sugar? Home economics journalism currently is called consumer economics communications. A specialty within consumer economics may be nutrition communications or nutrition journalism. Usually a program of study combines all the courses needed to become a registered dietitian or consumer economist with courses needed to find work in journalism, public relations, advertising, education, or corporate and marketing communications. Look at the Web site for the Council for Responsible Nutrition at: http://www.crnusa.org/. It's about the science behind the supplements.

Shifting to another topic—attention deficit disorder—do you know what nutrients and essential fatty acids help to manage attention deficit hyperactivity disorder? Would it interest you to write a feature article, organize a debate, or develop a term paper on any subject related to nutrition, diets, lifestyles, obesity, diabetes, and other health issues, or consumer economics communications?

"Nutraceuticals (often referred to as phytochemicals or functional foods) are natural, bioactive chemical compounds that have health promoting, disease preventing or medicinal properties," according to the definition on the Web site of the Nutraceuticals Institute (Rutgers/St John's University partnership) at: http://foodsci.rutgers.edu/nci/.

Can you write about or debate issues and controversies on the health benefits of phytocompounds? Examples of phytocompounds include quercetin and resveratrol. Can you find the words 'phytocompounds' and 'polyphons' in your dictionary? Explain to the public the uses of food supplements sold in health food stores called 'quercetin' and 'resveratrol?' Can you define these terms to the general public in a magazine, news article, debate, or term paper on the credibility of the studies regarding the health benefits of grape seed extract?

Do you first turn to the research institutes on food or nutraceuticals for answers or search the alternative magazines aimed at the general consumer of health products? Or do you go to the research published in medical journals and compare the abstracts, studies, and reviews?

How do you explain the reduced cardiovascular risk and similar benefits of the latest nutrition-related research? Can you write in plain language for a magazine or newspaper how fish rich in omega-3 fatty acids, olive oil polyphons, and fruits, vegetables or herbs offers specific health benefits? If you're thinking about a career in consumer communications or nutrition journalism, what's the future outlook in a world of shrinking newspapers and downsizing of reporters?

Can the smaller, alternative media pay you enough as a journalist? Or should you become a registered dietician before you attempt journalism or other communications careers in food, nutrition, agriculture, or consumer-related areas?

Can you easily transfer your skills to medical, technical, and pharmaceutical copywriting with a background in journalism and the life sciences or nutrition? Which path is best to take to enter a career in consumer communications or nutrition journalism, a degree in journalism, nutrition, nursing, medical writing, or agriculture? Some universities do offer a degree in a major titled "consumer communications" or "nutrition journalism."

Would you have a better chance of finding a tenured career by majoring in one of the life sciences, such as ethnobotany or even medical anthropology? If you're interested in studying or writing about childhood or adolescent obesity, would a counseling psychology degree be the right choice?

Or would you be fully prepared only by attending medical school? Would nursing school be the right path for a career as a nurse practitioner specializing in obesity issues? Perhaps majoring in nutrition, becoming a registered dietician with a minor in journalism is the best focus to enter the world of communications with a specialty. These are but a few of the issues and controversies surrounding the evolving field of nutrition as a career.

Where do you find jobs writing about nutrition or consumer science, and what's the future outlook for this career? Or if you're a student interested in finding information to write a term paper or participate in a debate on nutrition controversies and obesity issues, where do you begin looking for information you can understand?

Who regulates dietary supplements? Maybe you only want to know enough about nutrition to participate in a debate or write a thesis or term paper for middle school, high school, or any university level from undergraduate to graduate. Perhaps you're writing a thesis on one aspect of nutrition or obesity. How do you narrow down the possibilities to one topic, find resources, and organize your project?

Where do you go to find out whether waist size predicts diabetes risk in men? What's the latest news on tomatoes protecting against heart failure? Is it true that cranberries improve the use of damaged blood vessels? Where do you find this type of news? The answer is in alternative magazines that focus on global health and medical findings.

Here's a guidebook for you to begin organizing a term paper, a debate, or a career in nutrition journalism and consumer communications. Gather resource material and ideas to write your term paper or organize your debate if you're a student at any level, librarian, or educator. Your goal as a nutrition journalist is to find out whether beneficial effects have been shown in credible published and prestigious studies.

This book is a debater's resource and a term paper or thesis research guide to current controversial debates on nutrition & childhood/adolescent obesity for students, librarians, & educators at all levels—middle school through graduate school. Here's your resource for making more informed decisions on nutrition and adolescent obesity issues, careers in nutrition journalism, and the world of investigative consumer communications.

You can use this book to decide whether you want a career in nutrition journalism or consumer communications. Or you can let the information guide you to develop your debate, speech, term paper, or thesis on any of the nutrition issues, obesity issues, or journalism career issues in the field of consumer communications, nutrition and food journalism, or obesity issues and nutrition controversies.

The main point of this book for librarians, educators, students, and parents is that the world of alternative publishing is growing. And one of its most important segments emphasizes investigative journalism on health research.

What are the latest news stories, controversies, and studies regarding health care, food/nutrition, and obesity issues? What findings are so new the media hasn't touched it yet? How do you interpret complex medical journal articles in plain language?

How do you separate food misinformation from truth in the media? What's the present and future outlook for a career in nutrition journalism, consumer economics, science writing, or consumer communications?

How would you organize and write a feature article for a freelance submission to a publication aimed at specific age or occupational groups such as the following: children, adolescents, parents, older adults, gerontologists, librarians, child development specialists, caregivers, middle school, high-school, and university librarians, instructors, public relations specialists, or other media and corporate communications professionals?

How do you support or critique the new *Food Pyramid?* And how do you interview nutrition professionals and physicians to detail substantiated health benefits?

What's the best way to research, organize, and write an article, term paper, or speech for debating intended for an audience with no science or nutrition background other than what's presented in the mass media? What resources can separate myth from fact when you need to discuss, write, or broadcast on the topics of nutrition, health, and consumer economics communications?

◆   ◆   ◆

Adolescent and Childhood Obesity: Controversies for Debate or News

How well do you present to others proven benefits for maintaining or correcting health problems related to nutrition or consumer economics communications? Are you contemplating a career in nutrition communications, medical journalism, or consumer studies?

Are you a librarian, teacher, or student researching nutrition-related topics to debate or to write term papers? Are you a journalist writing about food, health, or consumer news? The widely disseminated Food Pyramid in the news is updated regularly. The *Food Guide Pyramid*, which was updated in April 2005 by the

United States Department of Agriculture, is now called the *MyPyramid Food Guidance System*. Visit http://www.mypyramid.gov for updates of information.

Perhaps you have to organize and communicate details about childhood or adolescent obesity, diabetes, or nutrition-related controversies, research, or issues such as diet fads. Do you need definitions of nutrition-related terms? The International Food Information Council's *Glossary of Food-Related Terms* is included in this book.

Are you planning to write resource guides that students and librarians can use to research or organize term papers, debates, or learning materials? Consider first reading news releases intended for the media. They guide you to the original medical journal articles. The news releases also are written in the plain language you read in newspapers. News releases describe the outcome of research.

These nutrition, health, or science-related news releases are online and can be accessed by the public. It's a first step in learning how to interpret what is studied and reported in scientific and medical journal articles. News releases are written at the reading level intended for general consumer magazines.

To begin developing a news feature or magazine article, let's choose the topic of obesity and see how it is presented in the media compared to how the topic is reported in scientific journals. Most newspapers write at the fifth-grade reading level. Magazines vary, but those intended for general consumers feature material written and fifth-to-eighth-grade reading levels.

Obesity issues, debates, and controversies involve cultural factors, genetics, lifestyle, and eating habits. If the obesity epidemic worldwide affects more than 300 million people, why does the USA have higher obesity rates than most other parts of the globe? Is it due to having more TV and radio advertising devoted to foods? Having more fast food eating places?

Are there fewer safe places to walk in lower-income neighborhoods? Or could it be the emphasis on eating food higher in calories and lower in fiber? The effects are seen in higher type 2 diabetes rates in children, particularly Native American children, more food misinformation in the mass media, and higher obesity with its startling health effects seen in younger children. What's driving the obesity epidemic among children and adolescents?

The North American obesity epidemic includes children, adolescents, new immigrants, their children, third and fourth generation descendants, and people who have lived in the USA for generations. Read the *Journal of the American Medical Association* (JAMA) study dated December 15, 2004 that viewed the relationship between the number of years immigrants have lived in the USA and the prevalence of obesity among those immigrants.

Only 16 percent of the individuals surveyed had been born in another country. These people were less likely to be obese than those immigrants who lived many more years in the USA. Did the diets and lifestyle change when immigrants came to the USA? Is obesity a result of assimilation as far as eating and exercising habits? Was it the stress of trying to fit in, create a life apart, or maintain the former country's cultural habits and customs? These are issues for debate or research.

The 2004 JAMA study used data from 32,374 people over the age of 18 who also were included in the 2000 National Health Interview Survey given by the US Bureau of the Census. After so many immigrants were interviewed in person, the issue remains as to why immigrants are more likely to become obese the longer they live in the USA? How do their food, lifestyle, and activities change or differ from the old country?

If you talk to numerous immigrant women, some will report that they feel unsafe walking in their own neighborhoods. It's a combination of the safety issues in the street, being approached by strangers, language difficulties, religious customs, and the appearance or cultural dress customs of the immigrant women. In some cultures, married women don't walk outside alone.

With immigrant men, transportation issues and work also come into play. Immigrant women may not be aware of health clubs, gyms, and exercise techniques outside their own cultural spheres. Some would be afraid to walk an hour a day in their neighborhood or ride public transportation to shopping malls alone, parks, or other safer places to walk.

People spending long hours inside viewing TV and snacking or working in sedentary tasks such as computer work, sewing, crafts, cooking, chatting, and studying have to deal with the effects of lack of exercise, sedentary habits, and overexposure to advertising on TV promoting high-calorie food. These events combine with lack of recreational outlets.

The children of immigrants have to deal with issues of whether to take lunch to school, eat in the school cafeteria, or buy snack food for lunch from the local school sundry store. Eating fast food snacks at a school store instead of the school cafeteria also is a problem for those who are not recent immigrants.

The issue is the lines in the school cafeteria are frequently so long, the student doesn't want to spend the entire lunch period standing in line waiting for food they find unpalatable. These children, like the immigrants are immersed in TV advertising for snack or fast food.

Most middle schools don't teach courses in nutrition to 12-year olds, even though there are many excellent text books around. Cooking classes may still emphasize making snack foods or white bread. And few newspapers give recipes using extra virgin olive oil on vegetables instead of butter.

One controversial issue is the public school's need for funds generating by the sale of snack foods by the on-campus middle school or high-school snack, gift, and sundry shop. These shops also abound on college campuses. Students frequently pass up the school cafeteria lunch to buy unhealthy snacks such as chips and soda at the school store.

Funds from the sale of these snack-food items go to support extracurricular activities at most public schools such as sports, drama, science, and debating clubs. Without the funds from snack-food sales, the school clubs eventually would close.

Another issue is with the quality of school cafeteria food. The food usually is too salty, fatty, and generally unhealthy. Salads use less nutritious, but cheaper produce such as iceberg lettuce instead of the healthier romaine lettuce, red cabbage, tomatoes, onions, spinach, and zucchini. Restaurant lettuce or spinach may be stored for long periods of time, eventually losing much of its nutrition value. Is childhood and adolescent obesity and/or type 2 diabetes caused in part by genes, eating habits, and also by the food students buy at lunch time from snack counters?

According to the Department of Health and Human Services, Centers for Disease Control and Prevention (CDC), its 2005 article posted at: http://www.cdc.gov/nccdphp/dnpa/obesity/, titled, *Overweight and Obesity* notes that: "During the past 20 years, obesity among adults has risen significantly in the United States. The latest data from the National Center for Health Statistics show that 30 percent of U.S. adults 20 years of age and older—over 60 million people—are obese.

"This increase is not limited to adults. The percentage of young people who are overweight has more than tripled since 1980. Among children and teens aged 6–19 years, 16 percent (over 9 million young people) are considered overweight. These increasing rates raise concern because of their implications for Americans' health. Being overweight or obese increases the risk of many diseases and health conditions, including the following:

- Hypertension
- Dyslipidemia (for example, high total cholesterol or high levels of triglycerides)
- Type 2 diabetes

- Coronary heart disease

- Stroke

- Gallbladder disease

- Osteoarthritis

- Sleep apnea and respiratory problems

- Some cancers (endometrial, breast, and colon)

Although one of the national health objectives for the year 2010 is to reduce the prevalence of obesity among adults to less than 15%, current data indicate that the situation is worsening rather than improving."[1]

[1]See this article titled, *Overweight and Obesity* at the Centers for Disease Control and Prevention's Web site at: http://www.cdc.gov/nccdphp/dnpa/obesity/. This site provides a variety of information designed to help people understand this serious health issue and the efforts being made to address it.

Immigrants and their children also have weight gain problems after coming to the USA. According to a press release from the Journal of the American Medical Society (JAMA) Archives Media Relations Department, Public release date: 14 December, 2004, the more time immigrants reside in the US, the more likely they are to gain weight. The article also is posted at the JAMA and Archives Journals Website at: http://www.eurekalert.org/pub_releases/2004-12/jaaj-poo120804.php. According to the press release, reprinted with permission below, the US population is becoming more obese, and that includes the immigrants and their children. The JAMA press release reads as follows:

Prevalence of obesity among immigrants increases with longer residency in US

The longer an immigrant lives in the U.S. the more likely they are to be obese, according to a study in the December 15 issue of JAMA.

Since the 1980s, the U.S. population has become more obese, according to background information in the article. However, little information is available about the prevalence of obesity among immigrants, the fastest growing segment of the U.S. population, currently comprising more than 11 percent of the total U.S. population and an even larger proportion of many minority groups. Immigrants generally originate from countries where the prevalence of obesity is lower than that of the United States, but adopting U.S. norms over time may lead to an increasing prevalence of obesity among this population.

Mita Sanghavi Goel, M.D., M.P.H., of the Feinberg School of Medicine, Northwestern University, Chicago, and colleagues examined the relationship between prevalence of obesity and years of U.S. residence among immigrants nationally, and explored whether counseling about diet and exercise may differ between immigrants and U.S.-born adults. The researchers used data from the 2000 National Health Interview Survey. Information collected included body mass index (BMI, measured as weight in kilograms divided by the square of height in meters) and rates of diet and exercise counseling.

Of 32,374 respondents (representing an estimated 201 million adults in the United States), 14 percent were immigrants. The prevalence of obesity was 16 percent among immigrants and 22 percent among US-born individuals.

The researchers found that the prevalence of obesity was 8 percent among immigrants living in the United States for less than 1 year, but 19 percent among those living in the United States for more than 15 years. After adjusting for age, sociodemographic, and lifestyle factors, living in the United States for 10 to 15 years was associated with a BMI increase of 0.88, while living in the United States for at least 15 years was associated with a BMI increase of 1.39.

The association for more than 15 years was significant for all immigrant subgroups, including whites, Latinos and Asians, but not foreign-born blacks. "To illustrate the impact, for a typical 5'4" immigrant woman and a typical 5'9" immigrant man this amounts to an excess 9 lb. (4.05 kg) and 11 lb. (4.95 kg), respectively, in addition to any weight gained due to aging or other factors," the authors write.

The study also found that immigrants were less likely than U.S.-born individuals to report discussing diet and exercise with clinicians (18 percent vs. 24 percent; 19 percent vs. 23 percent, respectively).

"In summary, immigrants appear to assume a similarly high prevalence of obesity as U.S.-born adults with longer duration of residence. With the growing immigrant population in the United States, early clinician intervention on diet and physical activity may represent an important opportunity to prevent weight gain, obesity, and obesity-related chronic illnesses," the researchers conclude.

◆   ◆   ◆

(JAMA. 2004; 292: 2860-2867. Available at www.jama.com)

Editor's Note: For funding and financial disclosure information, please see the JAMA article.

Another *JAMA/Archives* press release from the Archives of Pediatric Adolescent Medicine. 2005;159: 740-744, released on August 1, 2005, is available at www.jamamedia.org. The media release reports how waist circumference relates to insulin resistance in children and may identify children with cardiovascular disease risk and type 2 diabetes. The JAMA/Archives media release follows, reprinted with permission.

WAIST SIZE IS ASSOCIATED WITH THE METABOLIC SYNDROME IN CHILDREN

CHICAGO—Waist circumference is associated with insulin resistance in children and may offer a simple way to identify children with risk factors for cardiovascular disease and type 2 diabetes, according to a study in the August issue of the *Archives of Pediatrics & Adolescent Medicine*, one of the *JAMA/Archives* journals.

The prevalence of childhood obesity has doubled in the past two decades, accompanied by an epidemic of type 2 diabetes mellitus (T2DM) and potentially devastating cardiovascular disease (CVD) consequences, according to background information in the article. Some studies suggest that in adults, measurement of waist circumference (WC), an indicator of intra-abdominal fat, is a better indication of CVD risk than body mass index (BMI), a measure of overall obesity. Waist circumference is one component of the metabolic syndrome, a combination of health conditions, including type 2 diabetes, high blood pressure and high levels of lipids (fat) in the blood, that place a person at high risk for heart disease.

Valeria Hirschler, M.D., of the Durand Hospital of Buenos Aires, Argentina, and colleagues measured the waist circumference of children aged six to 13 years and compared waist circumference to measurements of components of the metabolic syndrome, including obesity (BMI), insulin resistance, lipid profile (fats in the blood, including cholesterol and triglyceride levels) and blood pressure.

Of the 84 children evaluated (44 girls), 28 were overweight, 40 were obese and 16 were normal weight. Statistical analysis showed that waist circumference was an independent predictor for elevated blood pressure, insulin resistance and elevated high-density lipoprotein cholesterol level. "In our study, there was a significant correlation between WC and all the components of the metabolic syndrome," the authors report.

"Visceral obesity may be an important risk factor for insulin resistance syndrome in children," the authors conclude. "Waist circumference serves as a readily available means to estimate abdominal obesity in the office setting. Normative data specific for ethnic group need to be collected. The present study showed that children with abdominal obesity, as determined by WC, have increased metabolic risk factors for CVD and T2DM."

(*Archives of Pediatric Adolescent Medicine.* 2005;159:740-744. Available to the media at http://www.jamamedia.org.) For more information, contact *JAMA/ Archives* media relations. E-mail mediarelations@jama-archives.org.

◆   ◆   ◆

Caffeinated Cola and Soda Beverages

For years, people have wondered whether caffeine raises blood pressure in older women. According to 12-year study of about 150 thousand women, researchers from Brigham and Women's Hospital in Boston and other institutions thought that caffeinated coffee increased the risk high blood pressure. Instead, the study revealed that "drinking soda beverages that contained caffeine, regular cola or diet cola, was associated with a greater risk of high blood pressure." According to the JAMA Report of November 8, 2005, the study found that coffee does not increase your risk of high blood pressure. But the news is not as good for cola drinkers. The study shows a link between drinking lots of cola and high blood pressure.

For women with an average age of 55, diet cola increased the risk of high blood pressure 19%, and regular cola increased the risk of high blood pressure 44%. It's still too soon to blame caffeinated sodas and colas for the increase in the risk of high blood pressure.

What you can do is read the entire study. Do research on similar recent studies. According to the media release: "For sugared cola, the increased risk" of high blood pressure was "28 percent for younger women and 44 percent for older women."

Regarding diet cola, "the increased risks were 16 and 19 percent respectively." For further information on this study, see the Journal of the American Medical Association (JAMA) Report for November 8, 2005.

How Do You React to Caffeine?

Are you healthy enough to drink caffeine in moderation? Or should you drink decaffeinated green tea instead of caffeinated coffee? What do your metabolism, autonomic nervous system, and body in general tell you about how you react to any beverage, food, or candy containing caffeine? Before you start drinking coffee, you would need to research how your individual body and nervous system react to coffee compared, for example, to green tea.

Now the question becomes, are you in good enough health to even drink a caffeinated beverage without serious symptoms? What does caffeine do to your immune system or your pulse rate? Check out how your body reacts to a beverage before you form the habit of drinking it.

Would you prefer herbal infusions, decaffeinated green tea, or tea to coffee or some other beverage, such as vegetable juices? What's good for you as an individual? The point is know how your body responds to what you consume and how you exercise. Lifestyle and nutrition go together. What's best for your immune system?

Do you have genes that are sensitive to coffee? Does coffee make you nervous or cause anxiety or panic attacks? Does your heart twitch when you drink coffee? How does your own central nervous system react to coffee or other caffeinated beverages, or chocolate which contains caffeine?

Do you feel angry when you imbibe caffeine? Or do you have the combination of genes that allow you to drink coffee without feeling symptoms? Check out how your body responds to a food or beverage before you indulge. How does your genetic signature react to a particular drink or food item?

◆   ◆   ◆

Obesity

If you're debating the topics of obesity and nutrition or are interested in a career in medical journalism or nutrition communications, you might want to research the connection between adolescent obesity, TV watching, and soft-drink consumption. The JAMA/Archives has a search engine allowing anyone to type in key words such as 'obesity' or "childhood obesity" and find several media releases corresponding to the various medical journal articles on the topic of obesity. If you want more information, you can then go to the abstract in the actual medical or scientific journal.

At most university libraries the actual journals are available to the public. You can read the published study and compare the media releases explained in plain language to the actual journal article containing scientific terms and statistics. The journal articles, written primarily for researchers and health care professionals, but available to the public, contain more details of the study. What are not in the medical journals, at least in the same month side by side, are rebuttals alongside the study—just in case any of the studies are flawed, and a credible, recognized scientist points out the flaw in a letter or article.

Current public health campaigns to reduce obesity and type 2 diabetes have largely focused on increasing exercise, but have paid little attention to the reduction of sedentary behaviors. When beginning your research by reading a press release, don't get the press release, which is news intended for the media, confused with the actual medical journal article or the article's abstract (summary).

According to a JAMA press release of September 8, 2003, the prevalence of obesity in children and adults has been growing steadily for decades. Note that the September 2003 press release regarding the study, reprinted below with permission from JAMA/Archives explains in plain language what the researchers reported in the September 2003 medical journal titled, *The Archives of Pediatrics & Adolescent Medicine.*

Television Watching And Soft Drinks May Contribute To Adolescent Obesity

CHICAGO—Researchers report a correlation between television viewing and soft drink consumption and obesity in adolescent students in the September issue of *The Archives of Pediatrics & Adolescent Medicine*, one of the *JAMA/Archives* journals.

According to the article, the prevalence of obesity has been growing at an alarming rate in both children and adults for decades. In children, the prevalence of obesity doubled from the late 1970s to 1994 and is it estimated that 25 percent of children today have a body mass index (BMI) above the 85th percentile and 11 percent have a BMI above the 95th percentile. The decrease in physical activity and the popularity of high-fat, high calorie foods have been implicated in the rising rates of obesity. Obesity is a known risk factor for many health problems including hypertension and diabetes mellitus.

David J. Pettitt, M.D., of Sansum Medical Research Institute, Santa Barbara, California, and colleagues investigated the prevalence of obesity among sixth- and seventh-graders and identified lifestyle factors associated with obesity.

The researchers studied 186 boys and 199 girls in the sixth and seventh grades from three Santa Barbara schools who completed a screening study. Three hundred nineteen students also completed a short questionnaire about lifestyle, weight, eating and exercise habits. Height and weight were measured for each student, and BMI was calculated.

Overall, 35.5 percent of the students had a BMI at or above the 85th percentile and half of these students (17.4 percent) had a BMI at or above the 95th percentile. The rates were higher among Latino students and lower among Asian students compared to non-Hispanic white students.

The researchers found significant associations between BMI and hours of television watched and daily soft drink consumption (both diet and regular soft drinks). For students who watched less than 2 hours of television per night, 26.2 percent had BMIs at or above the 85th percentile, and 47.1 percent of students who watched 3 or more hours of television per night had BMIs at or above the 85th percentile. For students who drank less than 3 soft drinks per day, 33.2 percent had BMIs at or above the 85th percentile, and 58.1 percent of students who drank 3 or more soft drinks per day had BMIs at or above the 85th percentile.

The surveys also revealed that Latino students watch more television (2.4 hours per night) than non-Hispanic white or Asian students (1.3 hours per night) and consumed more soft drinks (1.6 per day) than non-Hispanic white students (1.1 per day) or Asian students (0.7 per day).

"Our analysis indicates that increased levels of television viewing and soda intake are associated with a higher prevalence of overweight and obesity among sixth- and seventh-grade school children, and overweight can lead to increased risk of developing chronic health conditions, such as type 2 diabetes," the authors write.

"Interventions that promote healthful lifestyle behaviors such as physical activity and limiting high-fat, high-calorie foods and beverages may be effective in reducing both the prevalence of obesity and the emerging epidemic of type 2 diabetes in children," write the researchers. (*Archives of Pediatric & Adolescent Medicine.* 2003;157:882-886. Available at archpediatrics.com)

Editor's Note: This study was supported in part by grants from the Santa Barbara Foundation, the Santa Barbara Cottage Hospital Research Program, the Andrew H. Burnett Foundation, and the Venoco Community Partnership Program. For more information, contact *JAMA/Archives* media relations.

2

Historical Nutrition Issues—Fad Diets versus Nutrition Research by Scientists

What are the current most critical debates about nutrition issues and controversies? Are the most critical debates about hunger versus safer food or food misinformation versus obesity? According to Dean O. Cliver, PhD, Professor of Food Safety, University of California-Davis, "Insistence on a zero-risk food supply will raise the cost of food disproportionately and cost more lives than it could ever save. Further, ultimate improvements in nutrition still will not yield immortality. We need to deal with hunger, in America and the world, first. Over any reasonable period, not eating is more dangerous than eating."

According to the opinion of Manfred Kroger, PhD, Professor of Food Science Emeritus, The Pennsylvania State University, "the most important issue in nutrition today is the lack of nutrition knowledge by consumers. This in turn has triggered the epidemic of obesity in our society. It seems that some want to lay the blame for that self-created problem at the doorsteps of the food service industry, food manufacturers, and even agriculture. It is simply self-control and understanding nutritional principles that will help deal with over-eating."

If lack of nutrition knowledge by consumers could be the most important issue, then food misinformation also could be the most important current controversy in the field of nutrition. Childhood obesity and type 2 diabetes are big nutrition issues in the news. What's a big nutrition controversy? It's the debate about whether technology works for or against nature. The average consumer is told most often in the media that science (or technology) versus nature. Then there's the debate between nutrition and advertising.

Nutrition and advertising have an inverse relationship. Processed food, such as sugary cold cereals that register high on the glycemic index, and heat-popped snacks are advertised, but not unprocessed raw foods, except on a few satellite stations that cost money for subscription. Advertising in the mainstream media features drug benefits and side effects rather than food and vitamin or mineral-based health benefits of vegetables and fruits or wild fish from less contaminated waters containing the health benefits Omega 3 fatty acids.

The problem is, when fresh wild fish costs $16 per pound, people are going to buy canned wild fish for $2 or $3 not knowing whether the fish in the can contains more or less of toxins such as PCBs and mercury than the fresh wild fish on display in the upscale food store. Consumers want to know whether paying less money in a chain-store supermarket or paying more money in an upscale food store will result in products that affect human health differently?

Up for debate, for example, is the controversy over where you buy your wild fish versus farmed fish and how much you pay. Are you paying more money for food with fewer toxins? Is eating wild fish better for your health than eating farmed fish? Why or why not? These are current nutrition controversies up for debate.

Most people like to look at a nutrition time line to see at a glance what nutrition controversies entailed in the past, present, and what will be the next controversy or issue hot for debate by scientists, the media, and the public. You'll find books touting the Paleolithic Diet and other books cheering the vegetable, fruit, nut, and grain-based Neolithic Diet.

Medical articles warning of the dangers of homogenized milk available after 1920. And you'll find articles comparing whole fruit to sugary fruit juices. How do you make informed decisions about all the issues and controversies in the field of nutrition today?

Whether you are a parent, teacher, librarian, newspaper reporter, or student at any level looking for hot debates on nutrition issues about which to write, you begin with the basic controversy in nutrition. It's the competition between science and nature.

The issue is whether nature is better than science and technology. Is technology an overwhelming improvement to health and nature in general? Are chemical solutions to moral problems also an issue? Can science be separated from technology when it comes to food production and distribution? Should it be? Why or why not?

Underneath the umbrella of science is technology. Scientific research needs to be funded by big business and/or the government in order for scientific research to be done on a scale that earns it credibility in the medical journals that have the respect of other scientists and the credible media. Technology is the method by which science applies findings to production of food products for the public.

Food Misinformation Nutrition Controversy Debate

What does the average person do when a new study comes out saying that a food has specific health benefits, but then soon after, another study is released noting that the same food has negative health consequences? This type of debate has opened the field of nutrition to debate. What health issues surround studies of soy products, homogenized milk, and margarine?

How does the average consumer with no science training make informed decisions about what foods are healthy for each person or for all individuals? Would the average consumer benefit by a costly test to determine whether one's genetic signature is helped or harmed by ingestion of a specific food or medicine? Are those tests accurate? Such topics are ripe for debate.

The hottest controversy in nutrition today is food misinformation appearing in various popular media—newspapers, general consumer magazines, and the tabloid press. However, three equally important controversies in nutrition actually are science versus nature, childhood obesity, and the ever-increasing type 2 diabetes epidemic in children and adults.

According to the International Food Information Council (IFIC) nutrition/food safety staff, while there are nutrition controversies almost too numerous to mention, a couple stand out—food 'myths' (or misinformation) concerning the safety/health benefits of consuming fish and seafood, especially canned tuna; and continuing misinformation about the safety of low-calorie sweeteners, such as Aspartame. For further information, the IFIC's Web site is at: http://www.ific.org/.

On the site you can click on links to several IFIC-produced resources examining these controversies in greater depth. If you're a journalist or other media representative, the current *IFIC Foundation Media Guide on Food Safety and Nutrition* is available free to credentialed journalists (members of the media). It contains valuable material on the history of nutrition and is a comprehensive resource on a variety of food safety and nutrition topics.

The print edition contains backgrounders; contact information for almost 300 independent, scientific experts; and links to reference materials found on IFIC.org. The new edition brings together, in an easy-to-use reference guide, information journalists need to sort out increasingly complex food safety and nutrition issues.

If you're researching the field of the nutrition as a writer, reporter, or documentary producer, the Media Guide is a valuable place to begin obtaining your background and contacts to interview. Ideally, reporters writing about nutrition would benefit greatly by having a degree in nutrition journalism. Several universities offer degrees in nutrition communications.

The programs combine communications and writing courses with coursework leading to a degree in nutrition, internships in writing about nutrition for the media or dietetics internships, and qualifying in certification and by state exam as a registered dietician. At the present time, there are no licensing requirements to be a nutrition communicator, researcher, or reporter working in any branch of the media from public relations to writing columns or books. To be a registered dietician, you'd need a degree in nutrition or dietetics and a passing score on your state licensing exam to be a registered dietitian (RD designation).

The controversy asks the question: "Is science better or worse than nature?" What is meant by 'science' actually refers to technology—the chemical and mechanical solutions to problems or states found in 'nature.'

Another question arises: Isn't science really nature, and isn't nature science? Three such topics related to the history of nutrition as well as its current state are about the psychology, anthropology, and sociology of eating. The psychology of eating forms the basis of most historical nutrition issues. One area of nutrition called "the psychology of eating" historically has focused on topics such as the study of slow eating, fad diets, and why people eat by habit.

Let's first take obesity as a nutrition issue. Childhood obesity is an excellent topic for a student's term paper, report, or thesis. In fact, childhood obesity is the biggest topic facing health professionals.

In an email interview received here (with her permission to reprint) on October 10, 2005 from Dr. Marilyn Townsend, Ph.D., R.D. Cooperative Extension Specialist, Nutrition Department University of California, Davis, CA she explains, "I think the most critical issue facing health professionals including nutrition educators is obesity among children and adults in this country." The connection between nutrition and health trends is an area ready for debate.

"As health professionals," explains Townsend, "We have yet to find the magic bullet to reverse the trend of increasing overweight. Since the majority of obese adolescents become obese adults with a complement of chronic disease risk factors, impacting the obesity rates in children is crucial to the long term health of this country."

What Other Nutrition Information is Available to the Public Online?

A lot of information online is written by people who may or may not have degrees in nutrition research. Another debatable topic is whether those who write about nutrition need training in nutrition and writing or in nutrition and science, or whether those without training in nutrition need to have experts as partners or co-authors on their materials.

Take the debate between the milk industry, for example, and those scientists studying the effects of homogenized and pasteurized milk on human health. What alternatives do you have that aren't sweetened?

A few, but many vegetable alternatives to milk contain sweeteners put in to attract people to taste. Then there's another debate: Are sweeteners added for taste addictive? Are they put in so you will buy more?

How many unsweetened brands are available to the public? What are the effects on human health of drinking unsweetened soy milk compared to sweetened almond, rice, or oat (vegetable) milk alternatives? Are any scientists studying all these alternatives to milk regarding effects on human health? If so, why are the studies not in the general consumer media?

How Safe Are Homogenized and Pasteurized Milk and Dairy Products?

One of the most debatable controversies in nutrition today is about the effect of milk on health. Check out the various articles and informational materials on the Weston A. Price Foundation's Web site at: http://www.westonaprice.org. According to the Weston A. Price Foundation's Web site (with permission of Sally Fallon to reprint the following information from the Web site):

1. "Dr. J. C. Annand has written a series of articles in which he has advanced the theory that the increase in the incidence of heart disease was proximately related to the on set of pasteurization of milk. Different population groups were studied in various parts of the world. His theory is that the heat process of pasteurization alters the protein found in milk and as a result heated protein is responsible for the large increase in the incidence of heart trouble in citizens of western civilization, during the course of the past generation."

2. "Dr. Kurt A. Oster has advanced the theory that homogenization of milk is proximately related to the atherosclerosis which is so prevalent in citizens in developed countries of the western world. The reduction in the size of the fat particles caused by homogenization permits them to be assimilated into the stomach lining in a manner that was not contemplated by nature. When these fat particles along with xanthine oxidase get into the bloodstream the human system sets up a defense mechanism which results in the scarring of arteries."

Take into consideration the fact that you have debates or issues related to many ongoing studies of how milk affects the human body. Before you can take notes on the issue of what type of milk or nondairy beverage is healthy for the human body, you need to look at the most current medical and scientific journal articles from primary and secondary sources.

Another issue to debate is how much antibiotics and growth hormones are put in milk sold to the public? How does organic milk differ? Does organic, raw, or otherwise differently treated or untreated milk effect human health in different ways? These are questions for debates on nutrition. To begin researching the field for your own reports, papers, projects, documentaries, or debates, look at the campaigns.

Begin by reading about both sides of the issue to get a perspective on what the controversy or issue actually emphasizes. Remember that "A Campaign for Real Milk" is a project of **The Weston A. Price Foundation**, PMB 106-380, 4200 Wisconsin Ave, NW, Washington DC 20016. Also see another link at the Weston A. Price Foundation's Web site at: http://www.realmilk.com/whichchoose.html. Raw milk is compared at the site to Pasteurized milk in California. While you're taking notes, remain unbiased and look at all sides and scientific studies to get a handle on what's being researched and why. List the pros and the cons, the health effects, and the consumer requirements of a beverage product such as milk.

Then research whether health-related studies are being performed on 'milk' that doesn't come from an animal, such as rice milk, oat milk, and almond or hazelnut milk. That's not milk at all, but a non-dairy beverage used in place of milk. What's the effect on the body, the sugar content, and other nutrients in each beverage? Who's studying that particular drink? What's new?

Every decade, new definitive guides are published on many aspects of numerous foods. Is there really a definitive guide in the face of changing research findings about almost all foods studied as regards to effects on human health?

The Homogenized Milk Controversy

Is homogenized milk good or bad for the health of humans? What about Pasteurized milk? The nutrition controversy and issues regarding milk have been ongoing in the medical journal reported studies for decades. What do cardiologists and other medical and scientific researchers report regarding what happens when one drinks cow's milk?

What about goat milk? And other nondairy beverages such as almond milk, rice milk, oat milk, hazelnut milk, and other smooth beverages that taste good on fruit or cereal that are not actually milk at all? What happens when they are unsweetened, plain (sweetener added, but no flavoring), or sweetened, and you take a reading of your blood sugar level shortly after drinking the beverage?

Here is one article published in the Sept/Oct 2003 issue of the *Well Being Journal* by Rodney F Julian. You can also find the article online at the following Web site: http://www.wellbeingjournal.com/homogenized.htm. Below, with permission is the reprinted article.

From Well Being Journal Vol. 12, No. 5 ~ September/October 2003

Homogenized Dairy, the Dependable Cardiotoxin

By Rodney Julian

When the "Father of Modern Cardiology," the eminent physician Dr. Paul Dudley White, graduated from Harvard medical school in 1911, he had never encountered coronary thrombosis. As a practicing physician in Boston, on those rare occasions when a hospital had such a case, he and other physicians from the Boston area would gather to see this rare disease. Today, however, it has become so prevalent, that it threatens almost all of us, young and old. So the question is "What happened between 1911 and now to facilitate this change?"

Many studies show evidence that cholesterol is the major contributor. Autopsy studies show that in American soldiers from the Vietnam War, 75% had evidence of atherosclerosis and high cholesterol buildup. The average age was 22 years old. It was natural to assume that since cholesterol was almost always present, it must be the leading cause of atherosclerosis. This assumption has continued to today. Many diets prescribed today by physicians or by diet specialists completely eliminate cholesterol.

Cholesterol is manufactured in our bodies. It is so important to the integrity of the body that all cells contain it. It is found in high concentrations in the brain. In addition to its role in the conduction of nerve impulses, cholesterol has an important structural role, as well as a biochemical role in endocrine production. Cholesterol synthesizes male and female hormones.

Without cholesterol, vitamin D, which is required for calcium absorption, would not be synthesized. Bile originates in the liver from used or spent cholesterol and is essential for proper fat digestion. With all this evidence indicating the physiological importance of cholesterol, why would the body keep producing it throughout our evolution if it were eventually going to destroy us? It would seem that the human system takes adequate care of itself. Perhaps, we are not taking care of the system.

The answer to the discrepancy between needing cholesterol for survival and finding it in heart disease victims comes from Dr. Kurt A. Oster, cardiologist. After suffering from two heart attacks, he was inspired to research how the atherosclerotic process worked. He discovered that the enzyme xanthine oxidase (Xo), which is present in cow's milk (as well as the milk of sheep and goats), can be very destructive to heart and arterial tissue *when the milk is homogenized.*

In raw milk, both the fat and Xo are digested in the stomach and small intestines. They are either used or excreted. Xo is found in the liver of many animals, where it breaks down compounds into uric acid waste products. Humans have a natural reservoir of Xo in the liver. One of its chief functions is to destroy used plasmalogen (*in the liver only*). And there are barriers, which prevent Xo from entering the bloodstream.

When homogenized milk was introduced in 1932, we started to see increased atherosclerotic damage on a regular basis. Under pressure of 2500 pounds per square inch, at a speed of 600 feet per second, milk is passed through pipes and fine filters. This breaks up the fat particles and puts them in suspension like a foggy mist. The homogenized process encapsulates Xo into tiny fatty substances called liposomes. This protects Xo from stomach acids and allows it to pass through the intestinal walls and into the circulatory system.

At this point, while the liposomes are circulating in the blood, they are slowly burned up as energy fuel, only to expose the hidden core, which is in fact the enzyme xanthine oxidase. This dangerous situation is taking place *outside the protection of the liver.* Xo and plasmalogen cannot co-exist in one location. The liver, therefore, cannot store plasmalogen.

It can only process or destroy it. So now this freshly exposed Xo circulating in the bloodstream, with nothing to stop it, starts to destroy plasmalogen, which makes up 30% of the membrane system in human heart muscle cells. In autopsies of people who died from heart and circulatory disease, plasmalogen was completely missing. Xo was in its place. Arterial inner linings were completely eaten away. The resulting lesions had become hardened by the deposition of minerals. Fatty streaks and cholesterol had surrounded the newly formed plaque by this time.

The appearance of cholesterol created widespread speculation that it was the cause of heart disease and not the result. The Xo process is slow and effectively destructive. Most 10-year-old children who have consumed homogenized milk have some form of atherosclerosis. In the case of American soldiers autopsied after combat fatalities, some had arteries as brittle as clay pipes.

There is a very high correlation between countries that drink homogenized milk and atherosclerosis. In countries where milk is boiled for safety reasons before drinking, Xo is destroyed in the process. However, boiling will rob the milk of vitamins, change its organic structure and convert it to a putrefied mess in the bowel. In children especially, it can lead to constipation, chronic sniffles and colds, and tonsillitis.

It has become trendy for health-conscious people to consume skim or low fat milk, but that only slows down the Xo process slightly. Besides that, low fat milk products will cause someone to gain weight. Farmers feed their pigs skim milk to fatten them up before the slaughter. If you look at commercially prepared homogenized milk in supermarkets, most brands state that vitamin D has been added. Unfortunately, vitamin D enhances Xo activity.

Xo is not the only source of atherosclerosis, but it is a major contributor. People looking to improve their diet in a truly healthful manner would be wise to avoid all dairy products, except for those that are raw or cultured without homogenization.

◆   ◆   ◆

Author's note: Dr. Paul Dudley White helped President Dwight D. Eisenhower recover from a heart attack, which allowed Eisenhower to continue his term in office. Years later, while still practicing medicine in his 80s, Dr. White became my father's cardiologist.

Rodney Julian has been a writer and researcher for over twenty years on the topic of natural health and healing. He is trained in Neuro-kinesiology. His practice in energy medicine is based in Dallas and he travels extensively for consultations and house calls. For more information please visit http://www.fetalogos.com or email the author at RFJ@fetalogos.com.

Recommended Reading

My Life and Medicine, by Paul Dudley White, M.D., 1971

Food Is Your Best Medicine, by Henry G. Bieler, M.D., 1965

Homogenized! Homogenized Milk Exposed, by Nicholas Sampsidis, 1983

◆   ◆   ◆

----- Original Message -----
From: <u>Rodney Julian</u>
To: <u>Anne Hart</u>
Sent: Thursday, October 20, 2005 3:10 PM
Subject: Milk Article

Hello Anne,
I wrote the "Homogenized Dairy…." article for the Well Being Journal. The publisher of the Journal is Scott Miner. I spoke with him about your request, to use the article in your book. He is giving his consent. And as the writer, I also give you permission to use the article. The only request we both have is that you give full credit to me and to the magazine (Well Being Journal). If you have any questions, please email or call.
Regards,
Rodney

Rodney F Julian
<u>www.fetalogos.com</u>

◆   ◆   ◆

High Carbohydrates and Cataracts

According to the US Department of Agriculture, Agricultural Research Service, in a July 2005 news report titled, "*High Carbs May Boost Cataract Risk,*" High carbohydrate diets were linked with a greater risk of cataracts in a study of 417 women age 53 to 73. New details about the association between high carbohydrates and cataract risk have emerged from a study reported in the June 2005 issue of the *American Journal of Clinical Nutrition* (volume 81, pages 1411-1416).

Women who ate an average of 200 to 268 grams of carbohydrates each day were more than twice as likely to develop cortical cataracts, than women whose meals provided between 101 and 185 grams by day's end. That's according to

ARS-funded scientists at the ARS Jean Mayer USDA Human Nutrition Research Center on Aging at Tufts University, Boston, Mass.

The recommended daily allowance for carbohydrates for adults and children is 130 grams. Researchers analyzed eye exam results and 14 years' worth of food records collected from 417 women, age 53 to 73. The women, participants in the nationwide **Nurses' Health Study**, did not have a history of cataracts but were recently diagnosed with the disease. Cataracts are a major cause of blindness worldwide and afflict an estimated 20 million Americans. Scientists don't know what links high-carbohydrate intake to increase cataract risk.

One possibility is that increased exposure to glucose, a breakdown product of carbohydrates, might damage our eyes' lenses. (See this July 2005 news report at the US Department of Agriculture's Food & Nutrition Research Briefs Web site at: http://www.ars.usda.gov/is/np/fnrb/fnrb0705.htm#carbs.)

◆　　　◆　　　◆

What are the 37 Most Controversial Issues in Nutrition on Which to Debate, Research, Write, Speak, Teach, or Produce Documentary Videos?

1. Food Misinformation in the Media

2. Does the FDA Protect the Public?

3. Can You Blindly Trust Big Business, Food Companies, Prescription and Over-the-Counter Drug Manufacturers, Vitamin and Nutritional Supplement Firms, and the Government?

4. What's the Way the Public Thinks about Nutrition in Different Countries?

5. Can Your Diet be Tailored or Customized to Your Genetic Signature?

6. Is the Mercury in Canned Fish or Farmed Fish Safe to Eat?

7. Are your Amalgam-Silver Fillings Full of Mercury and Affecting Your Health?

8. What Can You Do About Childhood Obesity?

9. Are Nutrition Journalists Taken as Seriously as Licensed Nutrition Healthcare Professionals?

10. What Kind of Fats and Oils are Healthiest?

11. Does Homogenized Milk Scar the Inside of Arteries? What about Pasteurized milk?

12. Science Versus Nature in Nutrition

13. Is Bottled Water Safe?

14. Fad diets versus nutrition research by scientists.

15. Does a High-Carbohydrate Diet Contribute to the Formation of Cataracts in Women?

16. Taking Control of Health Through Food Choices, Activity, and Exercise

17. Sugar or Sweeteners Added to Foods for Taste

18. Genetically-Engineered Vegetables and Cloned Farm Livestock.

19. Putting in Perspective Scientific Reporting and Risk Communication in Health News Stories

20. Establishing Scientific Basis to Support Claims for Health

21. Reversals of New Studies Regarding Food Benefits

22. Newspapers Devoting Less Space to In-Depth Nutrition Reporting

23. General Assignment Reporters Having Not Enough Training in Explaining the Importance and Meaning of Scientific Research in Plain Language

24. Reliance By Media on Experts with No Knowledge of How to Verify or See Flaws in the Expert's Explanation

25. Reporting in the Media Differences of Opinion Within Scientific Community

26. Scientists Not Sharing Findings in Different Fields that Affect Nutrition

27. Reporting Functional Foods Providing Health Benefits Beyond Basic Nutrition

28. Food Labeling Issues (missing ingredients from labels such as 'spices' meaning MSG rather than a natural spice such as garlic powder.)

29. Claims of a developing relationship between components in a diet and the risk of disease, as approved by the FDA and supported by credible scientific evidence. (How large is the size of the body of research needed in order to confirm health benefits?)

30. Consumer confidence in the scientific criteria used to document health effects. If the consumer has no scientific training, what method is used to gain consumer confidence? Is that method verifiable? By whom?

31. Issues of Mad cow disease, prions transmitted from animals to humans, hog-related influenzas and pneumonias that people can catch, and avian (bird) flu which is transmittable to humans handling the birds or poultry. Dog flu is under scientific study.

32. Soy protein: Does it cause health problems or is it healthy and may reduce risk of heart disease? Does it help prevent bone loss? Or does it over stimulate the thyroid? Is soy milk safe to drink or not? What is the ongoing debate about, and what are the issues and evidence? How much soy should or should not be consumed for what types of health effects?

33. Food allergies affects six to seven million Americans, according to the IFIC Foundation Media Guide, chapter nine, page 1. What should be on food labels?

34. Too much added salt to processed, packaged foods and restaurant foods.

35. Too many added sweeteners to processed, packaged foods and restaurant foods.

36. Trans-Fats added to packaged, processed, or prepared and restaurant foods and the issues regarding the effects on health of eating trans-fats.

37. World Hunger Versus Zero-Risk Food Safety for Longer Life and Improved Health

◆   ◆   ◆

Mangosteen in the News

Scientific research is ongoing on the fruit, Mangosteen. The fruit contains several classes of phytonutrient antioxidants, including a class of phytonutrients called Xanthones. As a communicator, what are the effects on human health of these ongoing studies of Xanthones? The health benefits have been observed for centuries where the fruit grows naturally in Southeast Asia. Some of these benefits have been scientifically documented.

As a journalist, your project could be to research the studies. Although no medical claim can be made for any particular food product, those interested in researching scientific studies on fruit can look at how Mangosteen is used in the French Caribbean and in Southeast Asia. What is the scope of the studies?

Investigative reporters who have an interest in ethnobotany can find out who is doing research, where the funding is, and how the fruit affects the human body. Does it protect against pathogens? If so, which ones? How do Asian healers use Mangosteen? What properties does the fruit have?

Is it expensive to import to the USA? Is it anti-inflammatory? Is it an anti-allergenic agent? Since no medical claims are allowed to be made about a fruit, how can you as a journalist communicate to the public what research is being done in what parts of the world?

How was Mangosteen used for the past several centuries? What type of folk medicine or folk nutrition surrounds Mangosteen in India, China, the Caribbean, Malaysia, and the Philippines? Start by contacting ethnobotanists, the USDA, and various ethnobotanical databases.

How is Mangosteen listed in the databases? Are benefits listed? If so, how many? That's how you begin research for communications, by looking first at databases. For more information, check out Dr. James Duke's Phytochemical and Ethnobotanical Databases Web site at http://www.ars-grin.gov/duke/. There's a disclaimer on the site that reads, "**WARNING**: Do not consult these databases unless you agree not to hold the compilers or host liable for any errors or omissions." The explanation reads: "Data were gathered rather randomly from the literature on economic plants, none of which will ever be completely known phytochemically." So here's a chance to practice your database research skills.

Noni Juice in the News

Noni fruit from Tahiti and Hawaii also is sold in health food stores and online and is being studied for health benefits. There's a book on the benefits and studies ongoing on noni fruit. It's titled, *Noni Juice: How Much, How Often, For What, 3rd Edition* by Neil Solomon, MD, PhD, 2000. Renowned medical doctor holding both an MD and PhD degree, Neil Solomon did an intense study on Noni Juice that comes from the tropical fruit Morinda Citrifolia. Dr. Solomon extensively surveyed 1227 health professionals representing over 25,314 noni juice drinkers from over 80 countries.

As a nutrition journalist, comparing articles in scientific journals to articles in popular media is excellent training for looking at the details as well as the big picture. (Yes, I drink noni juice as well as pomegranate and mangosteen.)

Each year or two, you'll notice, a new fruit is brought into the news based on scientific articles testing health benefits. As a journalist, your job is to reveal whether the tests were done on people or mice and let the public know whether the results apply to humans for each of the new fruit juices being introduced in capsule form or juice form or both.

Pomegranate Juice in the News

In 2005, Pomegranate *(Punica granatum)* made newspaper headlines. According to the March 22, 2005 National Geographic News article by Stefan Lovgren titled, "Pomegranate Juice Fights Heart Disease, Study Says," posted on the Web site at: http://news.nationalgeographic.com/news/2005/03/0322_050322_pomegranates.html, a new study done at the University of Naples, Italy, and at the University of California, Los Angeles, reports that antioxidants in pomegranate juice may help reduce the formation of fatty deposits on artery walls. Antioxidants are compounds that limit cell damage. Scientists used mice to test the juice.

The study revealed that pomegranate juice combats hardening of the arteries (atherogenesis) and related diseases, such as heart attacks and strokes. If you're a reporter with this story, you may be prevented from stating any medical claims surrounding fruit juice. And you have to reveal that mice ingested pomegranate juice. However, you would have to understand that it's the polyphenols [antioxidant chemicals] and other natural compounds contained in the pomegranate juice that may slow atherogenesis.

Read the scientific journal research published in the March 29, 2005 issue of *Proceedings of the National Academy of Sciences*. (PNAS 2005 102: 4896-4901; published online before print as 10.1073/pnas.0500998102.) See the article at: http://www.pnas.org/cgi/content/full/102/13/4896?maxtoshow=&HITS=10&hits=10&RESULTFORMAT=&fulltext=pomegranate&searchid=1131513392989_1916&stored_search=&FIRSTINDEX=0&journalcode=pnas. (Or go to http://www.pnas.org/.)

Compare the journal article to the news articles you see in the media. What was included or excluded to attract readers from the general public? Learning to write news about science and food requires reading the entire study and practicing to re-write the important findings. You'd need to find a scientist to interview who worked on the study. In the news article, the journalist interviewed Claudio

Napoli, a professor of medicine and clinical pathology at the University of Naples, Italy.

What the reader wants to know is why the fruit juice worked. You'd have to glean from the interview and from the original study the conclusion, that "The fruit juice is rich in natural polyphenols, including tannins and anthocyanins, which have protective effects on the arterial wall." But can the reader extrapolate conclusions on mice working similarly on humans? That's when the writer needs to get a quote from the scientist working on the study, such as Dr. Napoli's quote in the news article. Now the reader can jump to the conclusion that it's hard to transfer the findings to humans, but the quote included an amount—that "a pint of juice may have some benefit in patients with early stages atherosclerotic diseases."

You'd still need to interview an expert, look at the original study, and re-read the news article to get the big picture of how nutritional information is organized in a mass media publication—compared to what appeared in the original study appearing in the scientific journal. Scientists already know that polyphenols from red wine and purple grape juice can reduce LDL ("bad" cholesterol). But what the public wants to know is whether this antioxidant study shows that pomegranate juice can help to prevent heart attacks?

Readers already may know that the large, clinical trials on a variety of antioxidants have not prevented heart attacks and strokes, and that results on mice may not reflect the same disease in people. The models used in the experiment are important to consider. That's why interviews with scientists and physicians can help a journalist to understand what's involved in reporting health news related to food.

It's always best to read the primary sources of a study before you read the news article written based on the original study plus interviews. When you've done your own research, it's time to interview a scientist involved with the study who can give you quotes/comments that readers of mass media publications can understand.

3

Political Nutrition Issues for Debate

What Political Problems are Influenced by Nutrition, and how does Nutrition Influence Health and Scientific Issues?

In reality, nutrition-related decisions are based upon politics whenever *economic* issues expose conflicts of interest. Who governs and standardizes nutritional information and research in the USA? Is this question as ambiguous as asking who raises the price of gasoline? Politics is about responsibility.

The biggest political issue in nutrition is that the general public doesn't read the results of studies published in medical and nutrition research journals. And the terminology and ongoing results are not explained clearly in plain language in enough general consumer publications.

Viewing equally both sides of the issue, actually, the politics of nutrition refers to the internally conflicting interrelationships among people in a society who maneuver within a group to obtain power and control. The politics of nutrition emphasizes the methods, strategies, and tactics involved in managing, administrating, and controlling internal and external affairs of what eventually gets emphasized to consumers.

Theoretically, nutrition-related decisions should be based on impartial hard scientific evidence. Credible evidence is vulnerable to being shown to be flawed by additional research.

Politics of the Food Pyramid

The Department of Agriculture, for example, is in charge of designing and updating the Food Pyramid that appears all over the USA in most textbooks and publications on nutrition. The function of the Department of Agriculture is to promote the agricultural products of the USA and to offer guidance to consumers. Here, the issue and conflict of interest is caught between the responsibility of the Department of Agriculture to offer nutrition-related guidance and the Department of Agriculture's economic interest.

The conflict of interest is one of commitment. Is the Department of Agriculture committed to supporting its own agricultural-economic interests or committed to offering unbiased nutritional guidance? Who should be in charge of designing the Food Pyramid?

When a consumer looks at the new Food Pyramid, the first item noticed is the lack of guidance on what particular food items should be emphasized, and which items should be eaten in very small amounts. What's controversial about the new Food Pyramid is that information is missing about what foods should be eaten more and which foods should be eaten less.

A small figure that could be interpreted as doing exercise is added. Instead of what foods to emphasize, the new Food Pyramid now directs the eyes to a figure walking uphill. At first glance, the consumer may understand exercise is good, but how much? No guidance is given as exercise is individualized.

Which food items should be emphasized? This too, must be individualized, customized, and tailored to one's metabolism and even one's genetic signature—about which the average consumer probably would not immediately think when briefly glancing at the Food Pyramid. However, the mission of the new Food Pyramid is to give guidance on nutrition.

Another question is how does the Pyramid guide those on special diets? Economic trends are what influence the design of nutrition programs. Conflicts of interest between economic, political, and scientific forces may shape the design of studies, charts, tables, and research.

On one side of the issue, the Department of Agriculture is thought of by some academics and critics to be in need of a crisis public relations campaign because of its focus on nutritional politics and economics causing conflicts of interest. That main conflict is between giving guidance and serving economic interests.

From the other side of the issue, consumers see a new Food Pyramid emphasizing exercise instead of emphasizing which particular foods should be consumed in larger or smaller amounts. The main issue is: Should the same group that designs nutritional visuals offering public advice also be required to promote and publicize huge numbers of agricultural products of the USA? Or should the promotion of USA-grown agricultural products be handed to a marketing and advertising agency?

Other political issues in nutrition focus on the competition between vegetables and fruits grown in the USA and the competing proliferation of edible imports from other lands seen in the larger, chain supermarkets. Issues also include questions as to what pesticides that are banned in the USA were used in other lands, or what type of bacteria may be on the green onions or sprouts from a location commonly using human waste as fertilizer.

A division of labor appears to be what consumers hope will avoid those conflicts of interest. As to the new Food Pyramid, current information about what products and produce are healthiest to emphasize and in which amounts are what consumers and nutritionists would like to see.

Politics are dependent upon economic forces driving the various interest groups and agencies in power. Controversies arise when interests clash. Whether public interest groups clash over nutrition guidance or cultures clash over habits, behind the conflict of interest is the politics of economics.

Another important political issue in the field of nutrition is the debate about which types of food are healthiest. The food table published by the government's Department of Agriculture includes carbohydrates, fats, and proteins. The reason why fat becomes a political issue is because not enough information is provided in the newest food table published by the Department of Agriculture concerning which sources of proteins, fats, dairy products, and grains are healthiest.

Politics of Dairy and Calcium Consumption

For example, the food table emphasizes more dairy products. Three servings a day of dairy products are recommended. However, scientific studies are revealing that a diet high in dairy products (and also high in calcium) is not that healthy. In fact, studies appear in various medical journals showing high dairy intake is related to higher incidences of prostate cancer.

A Harvard study on the topic, published in October 2001, looked at dairy product intake among 20,885 men and found men consuming the most dairy products had about 32% higher risk of developing prostate cancer than those consuming the least. The link between calcium and prostate cancer suggested by the researchers reports that the more calcium a person takes in through diet, the less the body produces of a kind of vitamin D—calcitriol. And it is calcitriol that has been shown to reduce replication of prostate cancer cells.

There is no need for a very high level of calcium added to most foods. When milk is consumed, most people don't think of the hormonal factors in the milk and whether they are harmful or beneficial. Studies currently reveal that a high consumption of dairy products does not decrease bone fractures in older women. In fact, studies show that there is no benefit to a very high dairy consumption. People need moderate amounts of calcium. Most nutritionists and physicians emphasize that what you eat should be balanced.

Instead of loading the calcium, most physicians advise people to walk and take regular physical activity. Strength training is fine for developing muscles and building the upper body. Walking strengthens the lower body. With exercise, you may be less likely to fall or lose balance with age, especially when practicing exercises that build the ability to keep your balance—such as tai chi and chi gong slow exercises.

The main political issue surrounding dairy products and calcium requirements focuses on the heavy promotion of the dairy industry that dairy products help you lose weight. To the contrary, science has found out that there is a greater increase in weight gain connected with high dairy consumption.

You need calcium in your bones, not in your blood or arteries. According to Shirley's Wellness Café, a holistic health Web site at: http://www.shirleys-wellness-cafe.com/fertility.htm#bones: "In a 12-year Harvard study of 78,000 women, those who got the most calcium from dairy products actually broke more bones than women who rarely drank milk."[1]

The facts are that you need small amounts of vitamin K and vitamin D to help absorb calcium. Do you know what foods contain vitamin K and D or whether you need to supplement with small amounts of these vitamins as supplements—or what is too much?[2, 3]

Unless you can read and understand articles in scientific and medical journals, you are as general consumers of food, literally kept in the dark, and that is a political issue. Men also have bone fracture problems associated with high dairy consumption.

A 1994 study of elderly men and women in Sydney, Australia, showed that higher dairy product consumption was associated with increased fracture risk. Those with the highest dairy product consumption had nearly double the risk of hip fracture compared to those with the lowest consumption.[4]

According to the Harvard School of Public Health, "Each year, osteoporosis leads to more than 1.5 million fractures, including 300,000 broken hips."[5] Some nutritionists emphasize that consuming a lot of milk and other dairy products will have little effect on the rate of fractures but may contribute to problems such as heart disease or prostate cancer. On the opposite side of the nutrition issue is the dairy industry that promotes advertising stipulating that moderate dairy food consumption helps some people lose weight.

The final answers aren't in. An extensive list of the calcium content of foods is available online from the U.S. Department of Agriculture.[6, 7]

Most consumers don't read or understand articles in medical journals. If the mass media doesn't translate the data into plain language, the information doesn't get into the general consumer health magazines or the daily newspapers. For example, how often do you read in the news about how calcium affects your blood pressure?

Studies found that data are consistent with an inverse association between dietary calcium intake and blood pressure.[8] That means calcium in certain amounts had been found in that particular study sample to lower blood pressure. But too much calcium raises blood pressure in some people in that sample.

The size of the estimate, the observed heterogeneity among studies, and the possibility of confounding and publication bias indicate that an increase in calcium intake above the Recommended Dietary Allowance is not recommended at population level for the prevention and treatment of high blood pressure. How do consumers learn whether publication bias filters down to readers through the mass media?

The biggest political issue in nutrition today is that information in medical journals is not being given frequently enough to the general public—the consumer, and the scientific terminology is not understood by the general reader seeking health information because the average person isn't receiving information in plain language as to what is healthy.

Research and studies change as new information comes in. In 1980 foods touted as healthy in high amounts now are promoted as unhealthy in high amounts. Today, studies reveal the darker side of the effects of certain foods. The answer is a continuing warning that not all the facts are in yet and that nutrition research is ongoing.

Politics of Carbohydrates: The Glycemic Index

The Glycemic Index is a table of rapidly-absorbed carbohydrates such as cooked potatoes, white rice, and white bread. High glycemic foods have unhealthy consequences as they rapidly turn to sugar. Then insulin pours into your blood to reduce the sugar.

Thinking of the consequences of what you eat becomes a political issue when you consider the epidemic of type 2 diabetes among children in the USA today as well as increasing obesity in the population. Higher rates of stroke and heart attack also appear in populations consuming large amounts of white pasta, white rice, and soda. To combat the effects of high-glycemic foods is to replace them with whole grains.

Obesity among children and teenagers is a political issue when it relates to the proliferation of sweets, sodas, other high-glycemic foods in vending machines in schools and types of food in school lunches or snacks served. Also another political issue is concerned with the types of exercise outside of school or physical education in the schools needed to maintain health.

Type 2 Diabetes Epidemic in Children

Type 2 diabetes today is showing up in children younger than the age of 10 and in Native Americans. The political issue here is that the children are victims of the food industry's promotional campaigns and little exercise.

Calcium is being added to foods from orange juice to candy when there's no need for high levels of calcium added to snack foods or sugary beverages. The dairy industry emphasizes weight loss from eating three servings of dairy products a day, but nutritionists insist that such evidence isn't forthcoming—that there is a greater increase in weight with increasing dairy consumption.

Politics of Fitness and the Obesity Epidemic

Another political issue is whether lack of fitness is more or less important than what food is consumed. The reason why fitness is a political issue is because physical education classes in many schools are no longer required by law. Political issues focus on how much exercise is needed and what public schools now require in gym classes and at recess.

The obesity epidemic among children and teenagers in the USA has prompted studies of what young people eat and what types exercise they get. Excess body fat may be a greater detriment to the health of teens than a lack of fitness, a recent study suggests.

Findings from a study of obesity in teenagers, that was published in the July 2005 issue of the journal *Pediatric Research*,[9, 10] found that excess body fat in teens resulted in high levels of triglycerides and LDL cholesterol and decreased levels of HDL (or "good") cholesterol. Should physical exercise be incorporated in public and private schools as a mandatory requirement?

As civilization evolved, a reduction in physical activity ensued. Historically, the less time people worked physically gathering food, and the more they sat in sedentary jobs, the fatter they grew.

Walking now has become the most beneficial resistance training because it builds muscles and lowers insulin resistance. Studies now have shown that the number of hours spent watching television is related to the more obese you are. The average number of hours spent watching television in the USA today is four.

Politics of Trans-Fat Danger

Another important political issue in nutrition emphasizes the dangers of trans-fats. Several decades ago in the 1980s, food promotions focused on margarines. In the twenty years prior to the 1980s, studies focused on the high number of heart attacks and strokes attributed to the consumption of animal fats used in cooking with lard and butter.

Soon margarine replaced butter in supermarkets and restaurants. Baking release spray instead of butter became common in restaurants when frying omelets. The health effects of trans-fats had not been touted publicly in those decades. Emphasis landed on the bad health affects of butter and lard filling the arteries with fat, plaque, and cholesterol.

Around 1980, margarines high in trans-fats filled supermarkets and restaurants. Butter largely fell into disuse, replaced by partially-hydrogenated vegetable shortening and margarine. However, the high uses of margarines and hydrogenated vegetable shortenings only increased the stroke and heart attack rates. A trans-fat culprit finally had been brought to public awareness after another two decades passed.

Today, nutritionists tout the new, trans-fat free margarines available. What trans-fats do is increase the risk of inflammation, leading to heart attack and stroke. Trans-fats also increase the risk of type 2 diabetes. Yet more than 90 percent of the risk of type 2 diabetes is decreased by a diet high in fiber, exercise, weight control, no smoking, and not eating trans-fats.

Media reports include articles that recommend eating certain types of beans to provide the fiber which may help to delay or prevent the onset of type 2 diabetes in children, in some ethnic groups, such as Native Americans, and in older adults. Too often, the media reports don't refer readers to the studies and research behind the articles. Readers need to understand details of the studies published in medical journals. The media acts as a bridge so consumers can learn to interpret for themselves what studies reveal. There needs to be a better link between articles in medical journals and the mass media's interpretation of science into plain language.

Instead, mass media reports that healthful oil such as olive oil is recommended by most nutritionists. Can consumers be referred to a bibliography of scientific studies to read to check the facts or flaws? And who is the middle-person to correctly interpret the facts or flaws to the mass media in plain language? Who checks the facts in the mass media?

A balance of Omega 3 oils with other oils such as Omega 6 and Omega 9 are recommended by health-conscious nutrition professionals. The political point emphasized is that type 2 diabetes shows up today in an increasing number of children under age 10, victims of little exercise and aggressive advertising of the food industry.

Vitamin E Issues

Nutritional issues also surround vitamin E studies. Some studies reported that people with heart disease grew worse and had more fatalities and heart attacks when taking vitamin E at certain dosages. Other studies showed vitamin E did no harm when taken at lower dosages by people who did not have heart disease.

Early studies at first showed vitamin E reduced the risk of heart disease. For example, in the continuing Nurses' Health Study, involving more than 87,000 women, Dr. Meir Stampfer and colleagues at Harvard Medical School and the Harvard School of Public Health in 1993 reported a 41 percent reduction in risk of heart disease among nurses who had taken vitamin E for more than two years.

Atherosclerosis is inflammation of and hardening of the arteries by calcium, plaque, and cholesterol. Researchers in the continuing Nurses' Health Study reported that a beneficial effect of vitamin E on heart disease "is plausible because of the substantial evidence indicating the importance of oxidation of LDL in atherosclerosis."

In a 1993 study of women's consumption of vitamin E, reported in the New England Journal of Medicine,[11] "Women who took vitamin E supplements for short periods had little apparent benefit, but those who took them for more than two years had a relative risk of major coronary disease of 0.59 (95 percent confidence interval, 0.38 to 0.91) after adjustment for age, smoking status, risk factors for coronary disease, and use of other antioxidant nutrients (including multivitamins)."

The numbers referred to as the "confidence interval" which is defined in plain language as the expected range of outcome in the study, actually means that the results do not prove a cause-and-effect relation. Instead, the early study suggested at that time that among middle-aged women the use of vitamin E supplements was associated with a reduced risk of coronary heart disease. As the years passed, more randomized trials of vitamin E in the primary and secondary prevention of coronary disease were being conducted with a variety of results.

In 1980, 87,245 female nurses 34 to 59 years of age who were free of diagnosed cardiovascular disease and cancer completed dietary questionnaires that assessed their consumption of a wide range of nutrients, including vitamin E. The average vitamin E intake in the lowest-risk group was 200 IU.

During follow-up of up to eight years (679,485 person-years) that was 97 percent complete, we documented 552 cases of major coronary disease (437 nonfatal myocardial infarctions and 115 deaths due to coronary disease).

In that particular 1993 study, "further adjustment for a variety of other coronary risk factors and nutrients, including other antioxidants, had little effect on the results," according to the abstract of that New England Journal of Medicine article. "Most of the variability in intake and reduction in risk was attributable to vitamin E consumed as supplements."

The early 1993 vitamin E study with nurses didn't prove a cause-and-effect relation. Instead, the study suggested that "among middle-aged women the use of vitamin E supplements is associated with a reduced risk of coronary heart disease." Conclusions in the early study regarding public policy recommendations about the widespread use of vitamin E focused on waiting for the results of further randomized trials.

In 2005, a new study of the effects of taking vitamin E supplements appeared in The Annals of Internal Medicine appeared.[12, 13] The newer 2005 vitamin E study looked at 135,967 adults who also had previously participated in 19 studies.

Many were older than 60 years of age. Approximately 60% had heart disease or one or more risk factors for heart disease. Examples of some risk factors include smoking, a family history of heart disease, and high blood pressure.

What the scientists actually looked at were reported deaths in the 19 random trials and the dosages of vitamin E. These randomized trials compared vitamin E consumption with no treatment or a placebo. A pill or other medicine that has no effect on the body is what is called a placebo.

In order to find previous trials lasting more than a year that emphasized the effects of vitamin E, researchers also studied published medical literature dated until August 2004. The scientists wanted to look at the dosages of vitamin E and how the various low or high dosages affected the individuals.

The dosages in the trials varied widely—from 16.5 IU daily to 2000 IU daily. The next step focused on combining all the trial's data showing individuals swallowing different amounts of vitamin E. Finally, researchers looked at the death rate among people taking these various vitamin E dosages.

The scientists found that the consumption of 400 or more IU of vitamin E each day for more than a year actually increased the risk for death. For those individuals who took less than 400 IU of vitamin E daily for longer than one year the results were unclear and uncertain as to whether or not vitamin E increased the risk for death.

This conclusion left an uncertainty in the air regarding vitamin E. What some nutritionists now advise is that adults should not take more than 400 IU of vitamin E daily because it is still uncertain to researchers what the upper safe limit of vitamin E is.

The political issue for health food stores and those who sell vitamins is whether to sell or not to sell vitamin E containing more than 400 IU per dose.[14]

Currently, nutritionists may be divided on issues related to vitamin E consumption. Politically, manufacturers and retailers of vitamin E supplements are at odds with researchers as the trails and studies are continuing on the vitamin E issue. After several articles appeared in the mass media interpreting in plain language the results of the 2004 studies on the effects of vitamin E on mortality rates, numerous nutritionists focused on a rebuttal, claiming that up to 2,000 IU of vitamin E is safe.

Meanwhile, the rebuttals continue with nutritionists on both sides of the political arena. Those employed by the companies selling vitamin E will report the beneficial health effects of vitamin E. Nutritionists looking at death rates will report those findings.

Which side is right? Since the studies are continuing, safety is an issue, and all the trial results are not yet in. The issue is very complicated and constantly changing. There are no final results regarding vitamin E.

The question is whether studies were done for risk of heart attack among the studies of nurses or the studies of men? Were studies originally done on people free of heart disease and heart disease risks? How do the results compare with studies of individuals who had heart disease or its risks?

Another question is how did the medicines taken by those with heart disease interact with vitamin E? Were heart disease rates significantly lower in people taking vitamin E or higher?

Were the women studied totally free of heart disease before taking vitamin E? Was the total risk of heart attack mortality lowered by 24% in one study of vitamin E? The answers to all these questions are that the results are not yet clear. Also, what type of vitamin E was taken? Was it the d-Alpha Tocopherol vitamin E or Gamma type of vitamin E in the studies?

According to recent in vitro tests, Gamma-Tocopherol inhibits the COX-2 enzyme. Is it an important factor for a healthy cardiovascular system? Or is vitamin E only important in small amounts? Should the COX-2 enzyme be inhibited? Or does inhibiting it increase heart problems?

All these issues become political issues when the economics behind vitamin E sales and additives to foods comes into focus. Another safety issue arises from other medicines or supplements that also inhibit the COX-2 enzyme.

Is Gamma-Tocopherol a more effective antioxidant than alpha-tocopherol? Some nutritionists say that Alpha is better than Gamma. Nutritionists know that individuals get plenty of Gamma in soybean oil, which is quickly excreted by the body.

Research indicates that a ratio of gamma to alpha-tocopherol greater than 1:1 increases levels of both tocopherols in the body and that alpha-tocopherol alone may not be adequate to combat oxidative stress. Most consumers will not be able to interpret the research without some knowledge of how to interpret the results.

For example, some forms of GAMMA E also contain tocotrienols from palm fruit which provides high concentrations of all four tocotrienols: alpha, beta, gamma, and delta. In some forms of GAMMA E, sesame oil, rich in gamma-tocopherol, is used as the base rather than soy oil. That's why it's up to the mass media to interpret in plain language the results of scientific research that most consumers will not bother to research in the proliferation of studies reported in medical journals found mostly in university libraries.

The issues of where to find current nutritional information increase as changing scientific studies are published. As newspapers and magazines merge, and major media consolidates, fewer science writers employed by the mass media are interpreting the newest results for the layman.

What most nutritionists do agree upon is that the use of a good multiple vitamin containing folic acid and a mineral supplement is helpful, especially for women in the childbearing years. Folic acid in the recommended dosages reduces neural tube defects. Most nutritionists also recommend vitamin B12 for older adults.

Vitamin D is another issue because most people working inside don't get enough of it, and some nutritionists report that people need more than 400 IU of vitamin D. However, because the health risks of individuals vary, and some people have conditions, nutritionists cannot make a statement recommending any dosage of a vitamin or mineral for any one individual without knowing the health problems and risks of that individual or even how that person's body might react to a specific ingredient or vitamin.

Some nutritionists recommend iron for young women, and not for men. Other nutritionists don't recommend iron as it can build up in the body and contribute to heart problems, blood, or other organ problems.

When it comes to an ingredient found in spinach called lutein, some studies point to how it helps prevent the eye disease leading to the most frequent cause of blindness in the USA, macular degeneration. Other studies show negative effects of lutein.

On the positive side, according to a National Institute of Health (NIH) 1995 study, increasing the consumption of dark green, leafy vegetables appeared to offer some protection against macular degeneration. Researchers correlated the disease with dietary antioxidant intake in subjects participating in a NIH Eye Disease Case-Control Study.[15]

The investigators found that higher intakes of carotenoids were associated with a reduced risk of wet (exudative neovascular) macular degeneration. The carotenoids called lutein and zeaxanthin were strongly associated with reduced risk of macular degeneration.

These carotenoids are obtained primarily from dark green, leafy vegetables such as spinach, collard greens, kale, mustard greens, and turnip greens. Eating spinach and collard greens five or more times a week was found to noticeably reduce the risk of macular degeneration. The study showed vitamin E had negative effects, vitamin A (retinol) had no effects, and vitamin C derived from food had no effects on macular degeneration. Reports abound on the effects of too much vitamin A related to bone loss.

Issues in the politics of nutrition arise when press releases begin to disseminate to the general public and mass media. For example, On April 7, 2004 the North Chicago VA Medical Center issued a press release announcing that "lutein has been shown to not only help prevent, but to actually reverse symptoms of ARMD."

The general consumer began to buy up the lutein supplements without knowing whether there were any studies reporting negative effects or how much dosage to consume. Consumers can go to the Web site of the National Eye Institute[16] to view educational programs, statistics, data, and latest news.

What general consumers need to do is understand all sides of the issues. Without training in how to read and interpret scientific articles, consumers are in the hands of the general assignment reporter or science writer hired by mass media to interpret scientific facts in plain language.

About 30-33% of the members of the American Medical Association have humanities degrees, but not all science writers are members of the American Medical Association. There also are other professional associations that science writers for mass media publications belong to such as the National Association of Science Writers and the American Association of Journalists and Authors. Mass media science writers don't have to be licensed, degreed in science, or belong to any professional or regulatory association.

Consumers don't really know whether or not articles they read in newspapers or general consumer magazines are written by someone with training in nutrition, medicine, or in the science of understanding and interpreting the results correctly in easy-to-understand words of medical articles. Graduate degree programs in nutrition journalism are very helpful in turning out writers trained both in nutrition and in journalism—interpreting to the public in layman's language what scientific journals find. The proliferation of information changing daily is overwhelming, and that is the biggest issue of keeping up with the times.

For example, when looking at a medical article to see whether there are any negative effects of lutein, the general consumer comes up against terminology like the following excerpt from the article, *"Effect Of Simultaneous, Single Oral Doses Of B-Carotene With Lutein Or Lycopene On The B-Carotene And Retinyl Ester Responses In The Triacylglycerol-Rich Lipoprotein Fraction Of Men1–3."*[17]

"On entering the bloodstream, chylomicrons become delipidated by the lipoprotein lipase activity associated with the endothelium and with circulating plasma lipoproteins. The remaining chylomicron remnants are finally trapped by the liver through a receptor-mediated mechanism. It has been shown that the apolar carotenoids accumulate in the core of the chylomicron particles, whereas the more polar carotenoids are more likely found at the surface and are therefore more prone to exchange with other lipoprotein particles in the circulation ([17, 19])."[18]

Are general consumers expected to decipher the medical terminology and understand that carotenoids get trapped by the liver and accumulate? That's why people consult professional nutritionists to interpret the results of the latest studies, some showing the negative effects shown in recent studies of lutein. The main issue is how the consumer makes a decision based on weighing pros and cons as studies constantly are changing in the field of nutrition.

This study showed that lutein, but not lycopene, negatively affected beta-carotene absorption when given simultaneously with beta-carotene but apparently had no effect on beta-carotene cleavage. How would the general consumer know a pilot study was performed to evaluate "application of TRL response curves to measure absorption of carotenoids from vegetable sources (15 mg carotenoid as carrots, spinach, and tomato paste)?"

Information appears at the NCBI (Pub Med) Web site of the National Library of Medicine (Indexed for Medline). The articles all are available to the public for a fee, and abstracts of the articles are free to peruse by the public. So both physicians and the general consumer do have access to the latest and the older scientific articles and published research studies. The issue is about understanding the terminology.

What would the general public want to find out? Adequate intake of lutein is said to reduce the risk of age-related macular degeneration, but actual information for developing a dosing regimen is sparse.

Ever since mass media news features flooded general consumer magazines, health and fitness publications, and daily newspapers reporting lutein being of help in preventing and aiding macular degeneration, nutritional supplement consumers have been increasingly buying containers of lutein and zeaxanthin powders or capsules. A July 2005 study on the effects of lutein consumption published in the American Journal of Clinical Nutrition reports, "Lutein was well tolerated and did not affect the concentrations of other carotenoids. Long-term supplementation with 4.1 and 20.5 mg lutein as beadlets increased plasma lutein concentrations approximately 3.5- and 10-fold, respectively."[19]

With a continuing array of medical journal articles, anyone can find both positive and negative effects of lutein. For the general consumer, answers are confusing, but the studies continue. Before you take any supplement, find out what the latest studies say about the negative as well as the positive effects. Weigh the pros and cons. And find out how the supplement is excreted and whether it builds up or doesn't build up in any organs.

Regarding any nutritional supplement, look at negative effects and realize that some substances actually build up in organs. You have to look at all sides.

Most consumers will want to know the answers to the following questions about any nutritional supplement. Is the substance taken daily? Does it continue to build up in the body?

Will one dose stay in an organ for a long time? Will I be allergic to anything in the supplement? Does any supplement contain a stimulant that will change my heart beat or induce seizures? In effect, studies continue on many nutritional supplements, and again, the answers continue to change.

The Politics of Omega 3 Oils

Another political issue in the field of nutrition centers on the quality of Omega 3 oils. Are the oils contaminated with PCBs and mercury, or are they clean and fit for human consumption?

In a 2005 study of Omega-3 fatty acids on attitudes and intentions toward purchasing novel foods enriched with Omega-3 fatty acids,[20] the study concluded that "the promoters of omega-3-enriched foods would be advised to direct their promotions toward changing the attitudes of consumers about the effectiveness of the functional ingredient."

The researchers wanted to identify "...the nature, strength, and relative importance of influences on intentions to consume foods that are enriched with omega-3 fatty acids using the Theory of Planned Behavior (TPB)." They designed a cross-sectional self-administered questionnaire.

What nutritionists in general look for is the quality of omega 3 oils. An issue that has political implications is that fish around the world contain varying amounts of PCBs and mercury. Nutritionists and the fish industry both want to keep fish pure.

So much emphasis is put on mercury and PCB contamination in fish that it distracts attention from the real political issue: that there are more PCBs in chicken than in fish. Chicken are fed contaminants, but PCBs in chicken are not as widely publicized in the media as PCBs and mercury in fish.

Unless popular feature articles about PCB uptake in chickens appeared in major daily newspapers, few general consumers with no science background would be able to compare mercury and PCB contamination in fish to chickens like the article appearing in a scientific journal such as the one published May 31, 2005 in Environ Int. on the uptake of PCBs in chickens.[21]

Most nutritionists know that chickens have higher PCB counts than fish due to the contaminants fed to most commercial chickens. The average consumer rarely reads articles in mass media publications comparing contaminants in chickens to contaminants in fish.

These studies appear frequently in environmental scientific journals of which most people have never heard the name and not frequently in general consumer food, health, or fitness publications. Another political question concerning what nutritional supplement oils are safe and which have varying levels of contamination is who is publishing tables comparing the levels of contaminants in oils available to the public?

When it comes to chickens, emphasis in the media is on reports of cases of bird flu in different nations, but not mass media or consumer magazine reports on who is comparing organic chickens to the large, industrial/commercial chickens to see whether there is a difference in the PCB contamination from any variety in what the chickens eat? Contaminants in chicken has become a political issue due to the economic realities behind the large chicken-breeding industries world wide, the fast-food industries, and the large chain supermarkets moving chicken to consumers.

There also is a movement in the nutrition industry comparing white meat products versus red meat products. Studies focus on the effects on health of eating red meat compared to white meat such as fish, chicken, turkey, or pork.

Researching is ongoing regarding any links to diabetes from eating red meat and whether women or men are more susceptible to type 2 diabetes or whether metabolic syndrome and type 2 diabetes are related to general diet and exercise issues, a lack of GTF chromium traces in the diet, genetic propensity issues, and/ or all of these factors combined. Sides cannot be taken when studies are still in process, and the results are not yet in.

Politics of the Soy Issue

Another political issue focuses on the soy industry competing against the dairy industry. Most nutritionists still maintain that soy in moderation is not unhealthy, but soy in large amounts can have ill-health consequences. Soy stimulates the thyroid. The question is how much, and what effects are being researched?

Asian communities have eaten soy for centuries, but in small amounts, including fermented soy products. Asians aren't consuming huge quantities of soy burgers, or drinking soy milk in large amounts, making tofu smoothies using 16 ounces of soy mixed with fruits in blenders, or using salty textured soy protein as hamburger fillers.

Also, isoflavones from soy have been extracted and bottled to be sold as phyto-estrogens (plant estrogens) as a menopause aid. The effects of large amounts of isoflavones on the thyroids of menopausal women are still being researched. Again, results aren't in with conclusions, but numerous articles abound touting various negative effects of soy used in larger amounts than what has been used historically as part of the Asian diet.

Most nutritionists agree that soy in moderation is okay as long as you are aware of the phyto-estrogen compounds in soy that block the action of your own self-made estrogens. After menopause, nutritionists report there is a higher risk of breast cancer in soy consumers. Nutritionists and physicians report that soy consumed by the young can use it in moderation. Some nutritionists warn older women not to use soy after menopause, at least in large quantities.

Nutritionists generally warn that soy milk in large quantities (which is too large a dose). Nutritionists don't recommend consuming soy products in doses higher than what historically has been eaten in the general Asian diet. The soy story is complicated because it becomes an economic issue.

The milk industry is threatened by consumers in large numbers turning to non-dairy substitutes. Claims from the non-dairy supporters report that homogenized milk contains fat molecules so tiny that they pass through the arteries and scar them, producing lesions leading to plaque deposits and hardening of the arteries. Before homogenized milk became mass produced, prior to 1920, milk didn't have this effect, say the non-dairy supporters. On the other side of the issue, the dairy industry claims that skim milk is safe.

Studies vary from reporting milk contributes to ovarian cancer, diabetes, and heart disease on one side to the benefits of milk on the diary industry side. Studies vary widely, some showing less bone fractures in Chinese women eating some soy. Negatively, studies also recently showed an increase in Alzheimer's disease and dementia and more cognitive decline in men eating soy in moderation. The soy issue is complicated, political, economic, and medical.

An April 3, 2001 article appeared on the BBC News Web site titled "*Soy 'Cuts Alzheimer's Risk.*" Researchers then reported that "Soy may reduce the risk of Alzheimer's disease, especially in postmenopausal women."

Previous to that article, research in the media suggested that soy also reduced the risk of heart disease and cancer. What researchers looked at in the late 1990s focused on a three-year animal study that showed that chemicals found in soy, called phytoestrogens, appeared to reduce the number of protein changes in the brain that are associated with Alzheimer's disease. Around the year 2001, reports came in to the media revealing how phytoestrogens mimic the action of the female sex hormone estrogen. At that time, the results of hormone replacement therapy with estrogen were not yet in, and estrogen was thought to reduce a woman's risk for heart disease and osteoporosis.

Later, science found that hormone replacement therapy had no effect on preventing heart disease. Back in 2001, estrogen also was thought to protect against Alzheimer's disease. So as researchers from the University of Alabama at Birmingham examined the impact of certain types of phytoestrogen found in soy, known as isoflavones, conclusions were made that today have negative impacts. Also, the 2001 study was carried out on aged female monkeys that had their ovaries removed to mimic the effects of being in menopause.

By 2005, studies hit the news stands on how soy eating and cognitive decline in men are possibly connected. What the public didn't know is that the original articles were presented at the 1999 Soy Symposium in Honolulu.[22]

According to that 1999 Pacific Health Research Institute study reported at the Soy Symposium, poor cognitive test performance in late life was associated with higher midlife tofu consumption. An independent association of similar size and direction was apparent in wives of cohort members, with the husband's answers used as proxy for the wife's consumption.

Midlife tofu consumption was independently associated with low brain weight and with ventricular enlargement. Independent associations of more frequent midlife tofu consumption with clinically diagnosed Alzheimer's disease and with poor cognitive functioning among nondemented subjects were demonstrated.

Tofu consumption has been linked to cognitive decline in another article presented at the 1999 Soy Symposium titled, "*Tofu Consumption and Cognition in Older Japanese American Men and Women.*"[23]

The purpose of the study was to determine whether the consumption of tofu, an isoflavone-rich food, influenced cognition in men and women. A secondary aim was to determine whether tofu consumption modified the association between ERT and cognition in women. The article suggested that estrogen may have a beneficial influence on brain function.

Researchers used the 100-point Cognitive Abilities Screening Instrument (CASI) to measure cognitive abilities. Researchers also measured low, medium or high Tofu consumption. After adjustments in the study for age, education, menopause, and language spoken, data from a sample of female participants suggested that tofu accounted for only about half of the soy-derived isoflavones consumed by this population.

The study found that, "The cross-sectional data suggested that high tofu consumption was associated with lower cognitive scores and opposed the beneficial association between ERT and cognitive scores in women." The political issue here, concerns the fact that the longitudinal data suggested that tofu consumption was not associated with the rate of cognitive change in older Japanese American men and women.

According to the research presented at the 1999 symposium, "Tofu consumption did not appear to oppose the beneficial association between ERT (estrogen replacement therapy) and cognitive change in women." Looking at past studies helps to reinforce the need to look at present and continuing studies regarding any aspect of nutrition.

The political issues today include new findings that estrogen replacement therapy has been found to have negative effects on women with heart disease or its risks, and tofu is still in a major political controversy. More soy products are being manufactured, and the dairy industry is losing consumers to alternative beverages such as almond milk, rice milk, and oat milk not containing soy products.

Another unrelated study at Yale University in 2000 revealed that the cognitive decline that may accompany old age or degenerative diseases such as Parkinson's disease could be caused, in part, by a lack of estrogen.[24] You can see that there are political and economic issues that tie nutrition, hormone replacement, and age into issues that change frequently—almost daily as new studies come in and old studies appear to show their flaws. How do you make a decision?

By 2003, an article describing a new study appeared in the publication called *Science* revealing that in one clinical trial's result, hormone therapy increased the risk of dementia. Rebuttals ensued in the mass media. Meanwhile, thousands of women on hormone replacement therapy continued to eat high soy diets, pop calcium pills in high dosages, and take isoflavone tablets as touted by some food supplement vendors at numerous holistic health fairs.

Vegetarian restaurants sprung up following the popularity of some of the best-selling fad diets. Many served deep fried tofu dishes over brown rice and meatless loafs made from salty textured soy protein.

According to an article published on June 22, 2004 by the National Institutes of Health, titled, *"Estrogen-Alone Hormone Therapy Could Increase Risk of Dementia in Older Women,"*[26] older women using estrogen-alone hormone therapy could be at a slightly greater risk of developing dementia, including Alzheimer's disease (AD), than women who do not use any menopausal hormone therapy, according to a report published in the *Journal of the American Medical Association* by scientists with the Women's Health Initiative Memory Study (WHIMS).[27] The scientists also found that estrogen alone did not prevent cognitive decline in these older women.

Political issues connected food with menopause in the 1990s and beyond because the Baby Boom generation of 75 million faced the onset of menopause in a designated time span. Studies on menopause and decline now focused not only on hormone replacement therapy but also on cognitive decline based on foods consumed, particularly soy.

The dairy industry's major competition focused on soy milk, soy cheese, soy burgers, soy breakfast bars, and other soy products replacing similar products manufactured by the large dairy industries. Today, the dairy industry not only competes against the soy industry, but also against industries creating alternative beverages that look like milk. Consolidation of the diary industries as well as the alternative food industries and mergers also are taking place.

Small, family-run organic dairy farms compete against huge corporations that inject cows with antibiotics and growth hormones, some of which have similarities to estrogen. Both large and small dairy farms compete against the alternative beverage industries producing soy, almond, rice, or oat products.

Nuts are a Political Issue

Time shows how nutrition issues change. In the 1980s, all nuts were condemned by many nutrition professionals as too fatty for the average diet. Today, nuts have been found by scientific studies to reduce the risk of heart disease and type 2 diabetes.

Nutritionists no longer fear the fat in tree nuts. Most physicians and nutritionists now encourage consumers to replace sweet and salty snacks with unsalted nuts. Roasted nuts are recommended because the fungus that grows on certain nuts such as peanuts is destroyed by roasting. Raw peanuts may contain a fungus that could infect the heart.

A peanut butter sandwich that doesn't contain hydrogenated fats, but is made from pure, unsalted roasted peanuts spread on high-fiber whole grain bread is now thought of as nutritious and healthy. Other nutrition issues that have political implications include the French paradox.

Why do the French as a nation have lower heart attack and stroke rates than people in the USA? They eat just as much fat. According to nutritional psychologist, Marc David, one theory is that the French custom of relaxed eating triggers the parasympathetic response in the nervous system, resulting in optimal digestion.[28.] David also mentions that ritualizing mealtimes leads to weight loss. The French emphasize nutrition-dense, high quality food which helps control overeating.

The field of nutrition is wide enough to encompass not only physicians, registered dieticians, and nutritional genomics professionals, but also psychologists and counselors specializing in the psychology of eating. What areas many scientists are now studying in nutrition also focus on the effects on health of ethnic diets.

Diets being studied also include the southern Mediterranean diet that is rich in extra virgin olive oil. Types of olive oil are being researched for their effects on health. Spanish olive oil is recommended as best by numerous nutritionists. Some nutritionists are researching whether the French paradox may also be due to the quality of the abundant fruits and vegetables or fresh fish in the diet.

One area of study asks whether the French paradox could occur due to the frequency and the similar amount red of wine consumed on a daily basis? Could the paradox be due to the resveratrol found in the red wine that contributes to the health of the French? Resveratrol is a compound found in the skins of red grapes.

Health food stores currently promote and sell resveratrol as a tablet. It also is known as The French Paradox, and in Chinese medicine as Ko-jo-kon. Originally resveratrol came out of oriental medicine.[29] In the past, resveratrol was used as a component of Ko-jo-kon, a Chinese medicine used to treat diseases of the blood vessels, heart, and liver. Resveratrol has been promoted for several years as the reason for the "French Paradox"—the low incidence of heart disease among the French people, who eat a relatively high-fat diet.

The Politics of Antioxidants

Do antioxidants slow aging? The abstract from one article published in 2002, in French, titled: *"Antioxidants To Slow Aging, Facts And Perspectives"* reports, "Although current data indicate that antioxidants cannot prolong maximal life span, the beneficial impact of antioxidants on various age-related degenerative diseases may forecast an improvement in life span and enhance quality of life. The current lack of sufficient data does not permit the systematic recommendation of antioxidants. Nevertheless, antioxidant-rich diets with fruit and vegetables should be recommended."[30]

On the other hand, health food retailers and vitamin vendors often generalize in lectures at holistic health fairs that numerous soil studies show that the soil in many areas is too poor to provide enough minerals and vitamins in fruits and vegetables for human minimum daily requirements to maintain good health. Thousands of health food stores and nutritional supplement manufacturers retailing and wholesaling online also depend upon the sale of antioxidants such as vitamins, powdered grasses, and food products based on assumptions that the soil is too poor to provide the minimum daily requirement of vitamins and minerals required for health maintenance. The political issue arises: why aren't more studies of soil published in plain language?

Is it true that the soil is too poor anywhere on Earth to grow vegetables and fruits containing high-quality vitamins and minerals? Or do studies of minerals and contaminants in soil focus on specific areas of the globe? What the public needs in plain language are definitions and nutrient values of health foods.[31]

Nutrition education is a political issue that currently is focused more on childhood obesity and less on the quality or merits of, contaminants in, or absorption of vitamins, minerals, and nutritional supplements (nutraceuticals). Has any average consumer actually read reports on soil sampling?

Political issues in nutrition require research in environmental publications. Consumers need to understand how to apply the results of studies to make logical decisions and choices about what to eat and when to supplement.

Studies are ongoing. Political issues focus on how the average person can best put together a healthy diet without sacrificing pleasurable eating experiences. For further research, an excellent Web site is http://www.nutritionsource.org.

Below is an example of what the mass media needs to convey to readers, perhaps in an online publication or resource booklet because there is little space in daily newspapers or magazines not devoted to advertising sales to finance the publication.

What the average consumer needs is a list of notes to check the facts and flaws of any studies mentioned or summarized in the mass media about what studies on nutrition really mean. Such a list of notes could be put in a flyer or brochure/booklet and look like the following:

Notes

Political Nutrition Issues

1. Feskanich D, Willett WC, Stampfer MJ, Colditz GA. "Milk, Dietary Calcium, And Bone Fractures In Women: A 12-Year Prospective Study." *American Journal of Public Health*. 1997; 87:992-7.

2. Bischoff-Ferrari HA, Dawson-Hughes B, Willett WC, et al. "Effect of Vitamin D on Falls: A Meta-Analysis." *JAMA* 2004; 291:1999-2006.

3. Weber P. "Vitamin K and bone health." *Nutrition* 2001; 17:880-7.

4. Judyth Reichenberg-Ullman, ND, MSW, DHANP. "*Is Dairy Dangerous?*" Last updated December 06, 2000. Online at the Web site at: http://www.healthy.net/asp/templates/Article. asp?PageType=Article&Id=617.

5. *Harvard School of Public Health*. "Calcium & Milk: What's Best for Your Bones," 2005. Web site: http://www.hsph.harvard. edu/nutritionsource/calcium.html

6. *USDA National Nutrient Database for Standard Reference*. Release 17 Calcium, Ca (mg) Content of Selected Foods per Common Measure, sorted by nutrient content is at the Web site: http://www.nal.usda.gov/ fnic/foodcomp/Data/SR17/wtrank/sr17w301.pdf.

7. *The American Cancer Society*, ACS News Center. High Calcium Intake Linked to Prostate Cancer: Moderation is Recommended, October 26, 2001. The article also appears on the ACS Web site at: http://www.

cancer.org/docroot/NWS/content/
NWS_1_1x_High_Calcium_Intake_Linked_to_Prostate_Cancer.asp.
1-800-ACS-2345 (or 1-866-228-4327 for TTY).

8. Cappuccio FP, Elliott P, Allender PS, Pryer J, Follman DA, Cutler JA. "Epidemiologic association between dietary calcium intake and blood pressure: a meta-analysis of published data." *American Journal of Epidemiology*, 1995; 142:935-45

9. *Pediatric Research*, July 2005

10. *Reuters Health*, Aug. 10, 2005.

11. Abstract. "Vitamin E Consumption and the Risk of Coronary Disease in Women." *New England Journal of Medicine*, Volume 328:1444-1449, Number 20, May 20, 1993.

12. *The Annals of Internal Medicine*. Vitamin E Supplements May Be Harmful, 4 January 2005, Volume 142 Issue 1, Page I-40.

13. E.R. Miller III, R. Pastor-Barriuso, D. Dalal, R.A. Riemersma, L.J. Appel, and E. Guallar. "Meta-Analysis: High-Dosage Vitamin E Supplementation May Increase All-Cause Mortality." *Annals of Internal Medicine*, 4 January 2005.

14. Edgar R. Miller, III, Roberto Pastor-Barriuso, Darshan Dalal, Rudolph A. Riemersma, Lawrence J. Appel, and Eliseo Guallar. **"Meta-Analysis: High-Dosage Vitamin E Supplementation May Increase All-Cause Mortality."** *Annals of Internal Medicine*, 2005 142: 37-46

15. Seddon JM et al. *Journal of the American Medical Association (JAMA)*. 1994; 272: 1413-1420).

16. National Eye Institute. 2020 Vision Place, Bethesda, MD 20892-3655. Web site: http://www.nei.nih.gov/.

17. Henk van den Berg and Trinette van Vliet. "Effect Of Simultaneous, Single Oral Doses Of B-Carotene With Lutein Or Lycopene On The B-Carotene And Retinyl Ester Responses In The Triacylglycerol-Rich Lipoprotein Fraction Of Men1-3." *American Journal of Clinical Nutrition*. Jul; 68 (1): 82-9. 1998.

18. ibid. notes[17, 19.]

19. Thurmann PA, Schalch W, Aebischer JC, Tenter U, Cohn. W. Plasma Kinetics of Lutein, Zeaxanthin, and 3-Dehydro-Lutein after Multiple Oral Doses of a Lutein Supplement. *American Journal of Clinical Nutrition.* 2005 Jul; 82(1):88-97.

20. Patch CS, Tapsell LC, Williams PG. "Attitudes and Intentions Toward Purchasing Novel Foods Enriched With Omega-3 Fatty Acids." *Journal of Nutrition Education and Behavior.* 2005 Sep-Oct; 37 (5): 235-41.

21. Pirard C, De Pauw E. "Uptake Of Polychlorodibenzo-P-Dioxins, Poly-chlorodibenzofurans And Coplanar Polychlorobiphenyls In Chickens. *Environ Int.* 2005 May; 31 (4): 585-91

22. Lon White. "Association of High Midlife Tofu Consumption with Accelerated Brain Aging." *Soy Symposium. Pacific Health Research Institute.* Honolulu, HI.1999.

23. M.M. Rice, et al. "Tofu Consumption and Cognition in Older Japanese American Men and Women." *University of Washington, Seattle, WA. Department of Epidemiology and Biostatistics.* University of South Florida, Tampa, FL. 1999.

24. Journal of Neuroscience 20: 8604-09. 2000.

25. Science, Volume 302, Issue 5648, 1138-1139, 14 November 2003

26. *National Institutes of Health.* "Estrogen-Alone Hormone Therapy Could Increase Risk of Dementia in Older Women." June 22, 2004.

27. WHIMS. *Journal of the American Medical Association.* June 23/30, 2004.

28. Marc David. May 2005. *The Slow Down Diet: Eating for Pleasure, Energy & Weight Loss.* Healing Arts Press.

29. Mike Derrida. Ko-jo-kon. Web site: *Natural sources of Resveratrol.* http://www.nanotech.com.cn/CGI-BIN/hbv/messages/763.html.

30. Bonnefoy M, Drai J, Kostka T. "Antioxidants To Slow Aging, Facts And Perspectives." *Presse Med.* Jul 27; 31(25):1174-84, 2002. (French.)

31. Stare, F.J., Hegsted, D.M., Mayer, J., Geyer, R.P., Gershoff, S.N., Herrara, M.G., McGandy R.B., Kerr, G.R. and Antoniades, H.N. *Health Foods: Définitions And Nutrient Values.* Journal of Nutrition Education. 47(3): 94-97. 1972.

4

Food Safety versus World Hunger Debates

An excellent debate in nutrition centers on the excessive fears for food safety. Are there true or false expectations as to what improved nutrition can accomplish? I highly recommend reading these informative scientific journal articles if you're researching the topic of food safety for your term paper, feature article, or public speaking presentation for debate.

Debate the topic of how much fiber intake should be appropriate. For research, read and explain in plain language the scientific article published in the American Journal of Clinical Nutrition. 31:1111–1112, 1978.

Should we ban or limit, or demand labeling of certain ingredients? Which ingredients? Debate the use of artificial and natural ingredients used in the US food supply. Read the article in the *Journal of Irreproducible Results* 34(4):18, 1989.) View the article on a proposal to impose an extra tax on "healthy foods" to help pay for the care of the additional elderly people who will result. Read *The Grassroots American* 1(4):12, 1995). Highly recommended are the monographs published in the (1993, 1999) editions of the American Council on Science and Health's monograph, *Eating Safely: Avoiding Food-borne Illness.*

What you might want to debate on in the field of nutrition are the types of excessive fears of perceived risks in food and the false supposition that improved nutrition offers a path to immortality. What do improved nutrition gains offer in terms of health values?

Which facts are valuable and which facts are unscientific and elitist? On one side of the debate would be the great deal of hunger in America. On the other side of the debate table would be many of the proposals that are being taken seriously.

The debate could be about which proposals are most likely to add to the ranks of the hungry and which proposals are focused on safer food and better nutrition leading to longer life spans, improved health at a later age, or childhood health through nutrition.

Another debate for public speakers or students writing term papers could focus on the fact that at least one-third of the world's population lacks access to food on a regular basis.

You could debate the American quest for a zero-risk food supply (as evidenced by alarms over Alar, genetic engineering, mercury in fish, PCBs in chicken, or food irradiation. The other side of the debate question could emphasize what the cost would be in human and animal lives. Use statistics such as the fact that presently 4000/year of people die from malnutrition in the US. The opposite side of the debate table would be about how many lives are saved by focusing on a zero-risk food supply.

As regards the role food plays in the prolongation of life, for your debate or term paper subject, read the excellent, published 1990 essay proposing that the US build a National Institute of Natural Causes to employ the medical scientists who will be out of jobs after all cancer and heart disease have been prevented (FRI [Food Research Institute, University of Wisconsin, Madison] Newsletter, Vol. 2, No. 1, April 1990).

Your own essay or debate could be on the subject of what role food research plays in the cure for certain diseases or in making life spans longer and healthier. If all diseases were cured, who would employ all the researchers? Who would lose or gain an income? Think about these subjects for your term paper, debate, or public speaking presentation.

◆   ◆   ◆

Who Monitors the Mercury in Sea Food?

Reprinted with the permission of the International Food Information Council. Their Web site with this information is at: http://www.ific. org/publications/qa/mercuryqa.cfm. © 2005 IFIC Foundation

Questions and Answers About Mercury in the Environment and Food

---

August 2005

Q. What is mercury?

A. Mercury is an element and a metal. It's released into the atmosphere both by nature through mercury vapor that's emitted from the Earth's crust and through the burning of household and industrial wastes, including fossil fuels.

Q. How does methylmercury enter our food?

A. Mercury finds its way into the food chain when naturally occurring mercury (such as from underwater volcanoes) or mercury from air pollutants is deposited into rivers and lakes. Once in the water, bacteria transform the air-borne mercury into methylmercury. Larger, predatory species of fish, such as shark and sword-fish, absorb methylmercury from the water and ingest it when eating algae and other smaller species of fish.

Q. Besides eating fish, are there other ways in which humans are exposed to mercury?

A. Yes. There are several ways, but the most common has been through dental fillings (known as dental amalgams).

Q. Who monitors the levels of methylmercury in seafood?

A. In the United States, the responsibility for regulating mercury is shared by two federal agencies: the Food and Drug Administration (FDA) and the Environmental Protection Agency (EPA). The FDA regulates commercially sold fish and seafood while the EPA regulates the amount of mercury released into the environment and works with state government agencies to develop fresh water fish advisories for recreationally caught fish. These agencies have issued consumption advice for pregnant women, nursing mothers, women who might become pregnant and young children.

Q. How much methylmercury is found in fish and seafood?

A. Levels of methylmercury, measured in parts per million (ppm), vary greatly, largely based upon the species, size and age of the fish.

According to the FDA, in general, methylmercury levels for most fish range from less than 0.01 parts per million (ppm) to 0.5 ppm. The average concentration for commercially important species is less than 0.3 ppm. In a few species, methylmercury levels can reach 1 ppm, which is the limit allowed by the FDA in fish intended for human consumption. This level is found most often in large preda-tor fish, including shark and swordfish. Fresh-water species—such as pike and walleye (which are also predator fish)—sometimes have methylmercury levels in the 1 ppm range, if they swim in waters polluted with high mercury levels. A comprehensive list of <u>mercury levels in commercial fish and shellfish</u> is available from the FDA.

Q. What are the health effects associated with methylmercury exposure and who is at risk?

A. Nearly all fish and shellfish contain traces of mercury, therefore people can be exposed to methylmercury by eating fish. While most people's fish consumption does not cause a health concern, high levels of mercury in the blood stream can have an effect on the developing nervous system of young children and unborn babies. Therefore, according to the <u>2004 FDA/EPA consumer advisory on meth-ylmercury in fish</u>, pregnant women, nursing mothers, women of childbearing age and those who might become pregnant and young children should follow this advice:

The advisory currently states:

1. Do not eat Shark, Swordfish, King Mackerel, or Tilefish because they con-tain high levels of mercury.

2. Eat up to 12 ounces (2 average meals) a week of a variety of fish and shellfish that are lower in mercury.

    • Five of the most commonly eaten fish that are low in mercury are shrimp, canned light tuna, salmon, pollock, and catfish.

    • Another commonly eaten fish, albacore ("white") tuna has more mercury than canned light tuna. So, when choosing your two meals of fish and shellfish, you may eat up to 6 ounces (one average meal) of albacore tuna per week.

3. Check local advisories about the safety of fish caught by family and friends in your local lakes, rivers, and coastal areas. If no advice is available, eat up to 6 ounces (one average meal) per week of fish you catch from local waters, but don't consume any other fish during that week.

By following these 3 recommendations for selecting and eating fish or shellfish, women and young children will receive the benefits of eating fish and shellfish and be confident that they have reduced their exposure to the harmful effects of mercury.

Q. Why does the FDA recommend a limit for methylmercury exposure?

A. The FDA is conservative in protecting the health of American consumers. Since methylmercury can be especially harmful to the developing nervous systems of the fetus and very young children, FDA has set consumption advice at the1-ppm level. This is the limit allowed by the FDA for fish intended for human consumption. This conservative level allows for the greater protection of everyone—adults, children and unborn babies.

Q. What about freshwater fish caught by family and friends?

A. The joint FDA/ EPA consumer advice recommends that before going fishing to check your Fishing Regulations Booklet for information about recreationally caught fish. Local advisories are also available through your local health department. If no advisory is available, it is recommended to eat no more that 6 ounces of fish per week including fish caught from local waters.

Q. What precautions should women take to reduce these risks?

A. The FDA and EPA recommend that pregnant women and women of child-bearing age who may become pregnant and young children should not eat shark, swordfish, king mackerel or tilefish. For these consumers, FDA and EPA recommend eating up to 12 ounces per week, two average meals, of a variety of fish and shellfish that are lower in mercury. Five of the commonly eaten fish that are lower in mercury include: shrimp, canned light tuna, salmon, pollock and catfish.

Q. Are children at increased risk?

A. FDA and EPA advise young children along with others not to eat swordfish, shark, tilefish, and king mackerel, and to limit consumption of fish caught by family and friends to one meal per week.

Q. How can people ensure that their diets are safe?

A. The two main things consumers can do are to eat a variety of fish and seafood rather than concentrating on one species. The EPA also encourages recreational fishers to follow state and local government advisories about which waters to fish. This information is available from the state department of health and is sometimes found in your Fish Regulations Booklet, provided when obtaining a fishing license.

Q. Should Americans eliminate fish from their diets because of methylmercury?

A. No. Eliminating an entire type of food or food group from the diet is generally unwise from a nutritional standpoint. Fish is an important part of a healthful diet; an excellent source of lean protein, vitamins and minerals. In addition, research has shown that omega-3 fatty acids found in certain species of fish help lower the risk of heart disease and ease the pain of arthritis, among other things.

There are ways to decrease one's risk of methylmercury exposure without denying the good taste and healthful benefits of fish. What's more, FDA and EPA both acknowledge that seafood is an important part of a balanced diet for pregnant women and those of childbearing age who may become pregnant. A National Academy of Sciences report notes, "Because of the beneficial effects of fish consumption, the long-term goal needs to be a reduction in the concentrations of methylmercury in fish rather than a replacement of fish in the diet by other foods."

Q. What do health organizations say about the benefits of eating fish?

A. The American Dietetic Association (ADA) recommends eating 2-3 fish meals per week, and points to fish as a low-fat source of protein that may help lower cholesterol. In addition, ADA says that research shows a number of benefits from consuming omega-3 fatty acids, found mainly in fatty, cold water fish like tuna, salmon, sardines, mackerel and lake trout. According to the ADA, omega-3 fatty acids help make the blood less sticky, so it flows through blood vessels more easily and is less likely to form clots which can contribute to heart attacks and strokes. The American Dietetic Association's position paper on Women's Health and Nutrition (1999) also recommends consuming fish 2-3 times per week.

The year 2000 revision of the American Heart Association (AHA) Dietary Guidelines included a recommendation that people eat fish (including canned tuna) for heart health benefits. "At least 2 servings of fish per week are recommended to confer cardio protective effects," says the AHA. The guidelines also mention the beneficial effects of omega-3 fatty acids in fresh and canned tuna and salmon on other diseases such as inflammatory and autoimmune diseases.

Omega-3 fatty acids, found in these seafood products, are important nutrients in all stages of life. They are essential in brain and vascular development of infants and newborns as well as provide beneficial effects on the cardiovascular system in adults who consume higher amounts of omega-3 fatty acids.

Related Information:

- Fish & Your Health
- Fish 101: Health Benefits Explored
- Omega-3 Fatty Acids and Health
- U.S. Department of Health and Human Services/ U.S. Environmental Protection Agency: "What You Need to Know About Mercury in Fish and Shellfish"
- U.S. DHHS and U.S. EPA: Mercury Levels in Commercial Fish and Shellfish
- USDA/DHHS Dietary Guidelines for Americans 2005
- Women's health and nutrition—Position of ADA and Dietitians of Canada

For further reading:

AHA Scientific Statement: Fish Consumption, Fish Oil, Omega-3 Fatty Acids, and Cardiovascular Disease, *Circulation*. 2002;106:2747-2757.

Fish & Your Health

March 2002

PDF Version

There's no doubt that healthful eating habits contribute to a healthy body. It's been known for decades that heart health, weight control, illness prevention and overall body functioning are all affected by what we eat. For women, there's the added importance of eating properly when pregnant or breastfeeding, because another person is depending on you for nourishment.

Say "Yes" To Seafood

Although no single food alone can make a person healthy, eating more seafood is one way that most of us can help improve our diets—and our health. Many of the studies about beneficial omega-3 fatty acids focus on fish as the primary source. Salmon, sardines, tuna and even shellfish are rich in omega-3 fatty acid content, but increasing your consumption of all types of fish and seafood is recommended.

The American Heart Association recommends that you eat fish rich in omega-3 fatty acids twice a week in order to reap specific health benefits. The American Dietetic Association and Dietitians of Canada: *Women's Health and Nutrition* position paper suggests consuming two to three fish meals per week, along with a low-fat diet, for heart health. Although all fish aren't high in omega-3s, they still can contribute important amounts of these fatty acids if they're eaten regularly. The following chart provides a general overview of fish and their omega-3 fat content.

Omega-3 Content of Fish and Shellfish
Amounts are in grams per 3 ounce portion*

Finfish

Catfish, channel, farmed, cooked, dry heat	0.2
Cod, Atlantic, cooked, dry heat	0.1
Flatfish (flounder and sole species), cooked, dry heat	0.4
Pollock, Atlantic, cooked, dry heat	0.5
Salmon, Atlantic, farmed, cooked, dry heat	1.8
Salmon, Chinook, cooked, dry heat	1.5
Salmon, Chinook, smoked, (lox), regular	0.4
Salmon, chum, cooked, dry heat	0.7
Salmon, coho, wild, cooked, dry heat	0.9
Salmon, pink, canned, solids with bone and liquid	1.4
Salmon, sockeye, canned, drained solids with bone	1.0

Omega-3 Content of Fish and Shellfish
Amounts are in grams per 3 ounce portion*

Salmon, sockeye, cooked, dry heat	1.0
Tuna, light, canned in water, drained solids	0.2
Tuna, white, canned in water, drained solids	0.7
Tuna, yellowfin, fresh, cooked, dry heat	0.2
Mollusks	
Clam, mixed species, cooked, moist heat	0.2
Scallop, mixed species, cooked, dry heat	0.3
Shellfish	
Crab, Alaska king, cooked, moist heat	0.4
Crab, Alaska king, imitation, made from surimi	0.5
Crab, blue, cooked, moist heat	0.4
Shrimp, mixed species, cooked, moist heat	0.3

*Cooked without added fat or sauces
Source: USDA Nutrient Database for Standard Reference

Getting Some Fat, But Not Too Much

Experts agree that a diet based on moderation and variety is essential to good health. In other words, eating some of a wide variety of foods provides more complete nutrition and is more beneficial overall than a diet that relies on just a few foods.

The 2000 edition of the U.S. Department of Agriculture's Dietary Guidelines for Americans recommends that people "choose a diet that is low in saturated fat and cholesterol and moderate in total fat." Fatty meats and full-fat dairy products (i.e., whole milk and ice cream) are the major sources of saturated fat in the diet. Sources of unsaturated fats are primarily vegetable oils. Diets higher in monounsaturated and polyunsaturated fats lower "bad" cholesterol levels, while saturated fats increase "bad" cholesterol. Therefore, an ideal diet would be high in monounsaturated and polyunsaturated fats and lower in saturated fats.

Increase Your Omega-3s

Within the polyunsaturated fat category, there are two important subclasses of fatty acids: omega-3s and omega-6s. Vegetable oils are rich in omega-6 fatty acids, and most Americans unknowingly get plenty of them in the diet. On the other hand, omega-3 fatty acids, which are found in fish and shellfish, tofu, flax, nuts and canola and soybean oils, are generally lacking in our diets.

Omega-3s appear to have a positive effect on heart rhythm and according to one recent study, may even reduce the incidence of the most common type of stroke. In fact, on the basis of the current research, the U.S. Food and Drug Administration approved the use of a qualified health claim for dietary supplements of omega-3 fatty acids relating them to a reduced risk of heart disease. Another intriguing area of research on omega-3 fatty acids pertains to their role in brain and visual function, as some research suggests they may have a role in preventing macular degeneration, a common form of blindness.

Continuing research involves the role of omega-3 fatty acids and the immune system, and suggests a positive influence on rheumatoid arthritis, asthma, lupus, kidney disease and cancer, as well as promising research at the National Institutes of Health on depression.

Getting Into The Swim Of It

Adding more fish and seafood to your diet is easy. One helpful tip is simply substitution. Slowly try substituting fish for one or more types of protein, thus establishing a twice-weekly seafood routine. Easy ways to do this include incorporating tuna sandwiches for lunch and sardines for snacks.

Here are some tips to help you get started:

- Start slowly by substituting fish or shellfish for another type of meal each week. Once that is an established part of your eating plan, increase to two seafood meals per week.
- Salmon and tuna give "burger night" a fresh flavor. Use fresh fish steaks to form patties to grill or broil. Canned tuna or salmon can also be used for burgers or fish "loaf."
- Try marinating and grilling fish "steaks" such as halibut or salmon for a change of pace. Grilled fish kabobs are also a possibility with firm-fleshed fish.

- Check your supermarket for a wide variety of marinades and spice mixtures to use with fish. And don't forget that old classic, lemon juice, garlic and herbs.

- Have a couple of cans of tuna on hand for quick lunch or supper ideas. A tuna salad sandwich or a tuna and noodle casserole can be ready in no time. (Just go easy on the mayonnaise.)

- Consider a "seafood snack" of tuna or sardines on crackers between meals.

- Introduce fish and seafood to your children when they are young, so they get into the habit of eating it.

- Choose broiled, grilled or baked fish more often than fried, which is higher in total fat.

◆   ◆   ◆

Reprinted with the permission of the International Food Information Council. © 2005 IFIC Foundation. Their Web site with this information is at: http://www.ific.org/publications/brochures/fishbroch.cfm.

Give Seafood A Place On Your Plate

Seafood is enjoyed by people all over the world. Its excellent nutritional content, good taste, availability and value price make it a staple food for many people. What's more, fish and seafood are frequently featured at cultural and religious celebrations by numerous ethnic groups and tribal nations in various parts of the United States and the world. Explore the many varieties of seafood and expand your collection of fish recipes—you and your family's health will be the better for it.

Frequently Asked Questions about Seafood

Nutritionally, how does fish compare with meat?

Fish and shellfish are excellent sources of protein that are low in fat. A 3-ounce cooked serving of most fish and shellfish provides about 20 grams of protein, or about a third of the average daily recommended protein intake. The protein in fish is of high quality, containing an abundance of essential amino acids, and is very digestible for people of all ages. Seafood is also generally lower in fat and calories than beef, poultry or pork. Seafood is also loaded with minerals such as iron, zinc and calcium (canned fish with soft, edible bones).

Why is seafood a good food choice for pregnant women?

For pregnant and breastfeeding women, seafood makes good nutritional sense. First, it's a good source of low-fat protein—important when you're trying to get the most nutritional value for your extra calories. Second, the type of omega-3 fatty acid known as DHA is thought to be beneficial to the eyes.

Scientists have found that women who ate fatty fish while pregnant gave birth to children with better visual development. And, babies of mothers who had significant levels of DHA in their diet while breastfeeding experienced faster-than-normal eyesight development. Preliminary research also suggests that a diet rich in omega-3 fatty acids—DHA in particular—may help decrease the chance of preterm birth, thus allowing the baby more time for growth and development.

Is seafood safe for pregnant women?

Yes. Seafood, including fish and shellfish, is a nutritious and safe food for everyone. Eating a variety of fish and seafood, rather than concentrating on one species, is highly recommended both for safety and nutrition. The U.S. Food and Drug Administration (FDA) does, however, recommend that pregnant women and those who may become pregnant avoid certain species of fish (swordfish, shark, tilefish and king mackerel) and limit their consumption of other fish to an average of 12 cooked ounces per week.

The reason for this recommendation is that, while nearly all fish contain some trace amounts of methylmercury, an environmental contaminant, large predatory fish such as swordfish, shark, tilefish and king mackerel contain the most. Excess exposure to methylmercury from these species of fish can harm an unborn child's developing nervous system. The FDA also suggests that nursing mothers and young children not eat these particular species of fish.

Can I eat fish that my family and friends catch locally?

Yes. Fishing can be great fun, and for some, cooking up the catch of the day is the best part. For most people, eating locally caught fish is perfectly safe. However, at-risk populations like pregnant women, infants and children should be especially careful. Be sure to check with your local health department to see if there are any fish consumption advisories about fish caught from specific lakes, rivers or streams.

Many states have issued fish consumption advisories due to high levels of mercury in local fish and several states have also issued advisories for PCBs. Anglers and their families should consult the local fish consumption advisories. The Environmental Protection Agency (EPA), which regulates mercury in the environment, advises limiting consumption of locally caught freshwater fish to once a week for women who are pregnant, may become pregnant or are breastfeeding, and young children. Other members of your family should also follow the recommendations of your state or local health department regarding how much local fish to eat. This information is sometimes provided when obtaining a fishing license.

What You Need To Know

The beauty of eating seafood is that it allows for a greater variety of foods in your diet. It's readily available, relatively inexpensive and provides nutritious protein and beneficial fat, which can ultimately contribute to a healthful diet.

It is important for pregnant women and women who may become pregnant to remember that the current FDA advisory on fish consumption provides information on methylmercury. Also, check with the EPA and your local and state departments of health for information on other environmental factors in species caught and harvested in your local areas.

Additional Information

Additional information about the benefits of fish and seafood in a healthful diet and issues relating to seafood safety can be found at the following Web sites.

American Dietetic Association
http://www.eatright.org

American Heart Association
http://www.americanheart.org

National Fisheries Institute
http://www.aboutseafood.com

National Food Processors Association
http://www.nfpa-food.org

U.S. Environmental Protection Agency,
Office of Science & Technology
http://www.epa.gov/ost/fish/

U.S. Food and Drug Administration
http://www.fda.gov

U.S. Food and Drug Administration
FDA Consumer Advisory
http://vm.cfsan.fda.gov/~dms/admehg.html

U.S. Food and Drug Administration,
Seafood Information and Resources
http://www.cfsan.fda.gov/seafood1.html

U.S. Tuna Foundation
http://www.tunafacts.com

Produced by:

International Food Information Council Foundation
1100 Connecticut Avenue, NW
Suite 430
Washington, DC 20036
http://ific.org

The American Academy of Family Physicians Foundation has favorably reviewed
this material through 2004. Favorable review means that medical information is
accurate, but does not imply endorsement of any conclusions presented.

◆   ◆   ◆

General Food Myths for Debate

Reprinted with the permission of the International Food Information Council. Their Web site with this information is at: http://www.ific. org/foodinsight/1999/mj/healthscaresfi399.cfm. © 2005 IFIC Foundation.

The Mouse that Roared: Health Scares on the Internet

Food Insight
May/June 1999

The World Wide Web is a tremendous resource for consumers and others who want an additional outlet to help them take control of their health. "The Internet is full of important, even lifesaving, medical information," stated Randolph Wykoff, M.D., M.P.H., of the U.S. Food and Drug Administration (FDA). But, not all Internet information passes the test of the Hippocratic oath. Enter: Doctor Deception who now makes house calls.

On occasion, some not-so-sound information spoils a wealth of excellent information on the Internet. With a click of the mouse, a word-of-mouth phenomenon can be multiplied exponentially via the World Wide Web or electronic mail and result in questionable nutrition, food safety and health stories being sent directly to your computer. In the age of the Internet and instantaneous global communication—in tandem with an increasing interest in nutrition's relation to health—it is not surprising that anyone with a modem can send consumers and others into a food and health panic.

Most of us have heard at least a few of the following myths that have been started and perpetuated on the Web: the great kidney harvest caper; the antibacterial sponge made with agent orange; the fluorescent lights that leach vitamins from your body; the cancer causing shampoo, and dozens, maybe hundreds more. These would all be simply entertaining if everyone recognized them as practical jokes, the mantras of unhappy people, or simply misunderstandings given life on the Internet. But not everyone can recognize these tall tales as fiction.

The Bias Belt

Some of the most egregious myths come from legitimate sounding individuals who have fallen in love with their theories. They believe they are serving the public by warning them of dire health consequences as the result of touching, smelling, eating or drinking a perfectly safe product.

Many consumers are confused and unwittingly oblige in the scam by forwarding the frightening electronic mail or referencing the site to family, friends and associates believing they are doing them a service. And, receiving one of these reports from a family member or friend adds to its alleged authenticity.

A recent *TIME Magazine* article (April 26, 1999) sums it up well: "The Web is praised as a wondrous educational tool, and in some respects it is. Mostly though, it appears to be a stunning advance in the shoring up of biases, both benign (one's own views) and noxious (other views)."

In most cases, there is no harm intended by those who position their opinions as facts. In other instances, the sly intent of the author may be relatively easy for health professionals, who have a strong science background, to detect. But, for some consumers with little frame of reference to tell fact from fiction, it can be misleading.

For example, an innocent Web surfer looking for information about dietary fats may stumble across one of several web sites spreading fear and confusion about a frequently used cooking oil. With a masthead featuring a skull and crossbones, or the headline: "Canola Oil: Deadly for the Human Body!" such sites may cause baseless consumer concern. If the consumer does not seek unbiased information, he or she will miss the real story: canola oil, a safe, monounsaturated oil, can help lower blood cholesterol levels when substituted for saturated fats in the diet.

Where Did You Hear That?

"At one time, doctors were the primary source of health information for consumers, but in the late 1990s the paradigm for securing this type of information changed," remarked Fergus Clydesdale, Ph.D., University of Massachusetts. Now, for both consumers and health professionals, the primary source of information is the news media. This information source replaces the traditional physician-patient relationship for consumers. For health professionals, media accounts now precede the medical journals and attendance at academic meetings. Often, a consumer first raises an issue with his or her health professional by asking about a story that ran in an on-line story, the local paper or on the evening TV news before health professionals have even received their journals.

A recent telephone survey conducted by Schwarz Pharma, Inc., and reported in the *American Journal of Public Health*, noted that approximately 29 percent of Americans have turned to the Internet for medical information—a number that, although not high compared to other media outlets, is likely to grow.

According to the *1997 Nutrition Trends Survey* conducted by The American Dietetic Association (ADA), 57 percent of consumers named television as their main source of nutrition information, followed by magazines at 44 percent and newspapers at 23 percent. Doctors and dietitians were at just 9 and 5 percent, respectively (see graph).

The same ADA survey, however, found that the tables were turned in terms of credibility. Information from doctors and dietitians/nutritionists was found to be "more valuable" (52%) than that from television news and newspaper articles (24% and 21%, respectively). The Internet may follow this same pattern of delivery versus credibility—the Internet or World Wide Web was found to be the least believable source of medical and health news according to respondents in the 1997 report, *Americans Talk About Science and Medical News* from the National Health Council. While the Internet can be a valuable source for scientifically accurate health information, it can also be a frontier town with no sheriff for assuring the truth of the information presented.

John Renner, M.D., of the National Council for Reliable Health Information remarked, "There is a health information shock factor on the Internet because there is so much information, both good and bad, marvelous and terrible. We've moved from a small library of information with a friendly librarian, to a huge warehouse with lots of people offering information," he continued. Consumers have not faced this situation before. The problem is the public can be deceived—believing that because they have seen something on the Web, it must be true.

A perfect example of how the public can be misled is a recent Internet article by a Nancy Markle that has taken on a "cyberlife" of its own. The article alleges that aspartame (a sweetener found in food and beverages) causes lupus, multiple sclerosis (MS) and other diseases and conditions, none of which has any scientific validity. Highly respected health professional organizations were fraudulently associated with the story, and numerous vulnerable people were needlessly frightened by this scientifically false allegation.

One of the marvels of the Internet is that as easily as you can receive inaccurate information, you can search for and find accurate information. If consumers were concerned about the alleged aspartame connection with MS, they could check the Multiple Sclerosis Foundation's Internet site for accurate information. David Squillacote, M.D., senior medical advisor of the MS Foundation wrote in his response to the Internet scare, "This series of allegations by Ms. Markle are almost totally without foundation. They are rabidly inaccurate and scandalously misinformative." Fortunately, numerous reliable organizations, Internet sites and publications have refuted this particular epidemic of hysteria and provided additional context for consumers.

The FDA's website is an excellent source for accurate information. Consumers wishing to counteract or confirm the aspartame story can find the following information from the FDA which could allay their fears: "After reviewing scientific studies, the FDA determined in 1981 that aspartame was safe for use in foods…To date, the FDA has not determined any consistent pattern of symptoms that can be attributed to the use of aspartame, nor is the agency aware of any recent studies that clearly show safety problems."

What's a Cyber-Citizen to Do?

How can consumers judge the validity of information received via electronic mail or popping up in a Web search? The foremost guideline for sorting the "trash" from the "treasure" is—just because something is printed on the Internet does not mean that it is true or credible.

Unfortunately for most of us, the best defense against nutrition misinformation and quackery on the Internet is in-depth scientific knowledge. Since not everyone has the level of scientific awareness or advanced degrees necessary to judge the validity of every story, the following tactics may be useful:

- Ask questions. Anecdotes and one individual's personal story are not scientific evidence.

- Look at the source of the information. A professional medical organization or government agency such as the American Academy of Family Physicians or the U.S. Department of Agriculture is more likely to have reliable information than an unknown person or group of people.

- If the story mentions a specific health condition, such as diabetes or breast cancer, search the Internet for reputable health professional organizations and foundations devoted to that disease. An example would be the American Diabetes Association or the American Cancer Society.

- Watch out for use of buzzwords like "conspiracy" and "poison."

- Don't take assertions at face value-give the other side of the issue the benefit of the doubt. Do your homework and call or e-mail appropriate health professional organizations to get a balanced picture.

- Consult with your doctor, a registered dietitian or other health professional.

The Internet has been a boon to consumers who want research and information on voluminous issues and topics at the tip of their fingers. It has also empowered many people to find health information to help them improve their well-being. Nevertheless, the ease of Web publishing has also given an unregulated forum to unreliable sources. Careful scrutiny and a healthy dose of skepticism are still necessary to determine what applies to you and what may need a second opinion. Internet sources for sound nutrition and health information

- Tufts University Nutrition Navigator
  http://navigator.tufts.edu

- The American Dietetic Association
  http://www.eatright.org

- The International Food Information Council Foundation
  http://ific.org

- Medline
  http://www.nlm.nih.gov/databases/freemedl.html

- National Institutes of Health
  http://www.nih.gov

- The U.S. Food and Drug Administration
  http://vm.cfsan.fda.gov.

- Mayo Health Oasis (of the Mayo Clinic)

  http://www.mayohealth.org

- Johns Hopkins Health Information

  http://www.intelihealth.com/IH/ihtIH

- World Health Organization

  http://www.who.int

- Food & Agriculture Organization

  http://www.fao.org

- Government healthfinder

  http://www.healthfinder.gov

◆   ◆   ◆

Look at the Year of Publication for Food Safety News

Reports and news published by the government several years ago may need to be updated. For example, supposed a food product is said to be safe in 1999 or some other year in the past. Then, several years later, the food product is found to be not so safe. That's why it's important to look at the dates. Take cooking oil for example. It may be safe in 1999, and it may be safe in 2006. Then again, there may have been new findings to show it is not safe. This can happy to any food or oil. I'm not saying whether it's safe or not because you have to do your own research and find out what's approved by the FDA and other government agencies.

What's a food myth several years ago may not be a food myth today, and then again, it may still be a myth. Find out by reading the latest updates of science articles in reputable medical and food science journals. Is canola oil safe today? Canola oil is not expensive and is found in thousands of commercial food products such as salad dressings and dips. Is Canola oil good for you?

Does it contribute to respiratory distress and changes in heart beat rhythms? Are there studies promoting the safety of the oil or any other health effects that are unsafe? Why does the oil remain in most foods you buy in the supermarket? Does it have beneficial health effects? Which ones? Compare the pros and cons of each type of cooking oil. How do you separate the food misinformation on the

Web from the updates of scientific research that may or may not change the news on any particular food or cooking oil?

Are the studies reliable and unflawed? What are the details? Is extra virgin olive oil, which is more expensive, actually better for you? To find out, do your research by reading the various medical studies published in scientific journals. Interview some unbiased experts that are familiar with various cooking oils. Are they working for the industry that manufactures the product? Are they neutral? Look at news reports. Read the latest research again. Decide for yourself.

Which Oil is Safest for You?

Before you decide on whether to use Canola oil rather than extra virgin olive oil, compare the safety of extra virgin olive oil, especially Spanish olive oil, to the safety of Canola. You compare by looking at the medical studies. How does Olive oil compared to Canola affect your heart beat/rhythm and respiratory illness? Look at the actual medical journal articles and studies for both types of oils.

See the Optimal Breathing ® Web site at: http://www.breathing.com/articles/canola-oil.htm. Look at actual medical articles rather than any personal opinions before you decide which oil is working better for your individual body. What are the results of medical research on these oils? What's the best way to decide what's accurate? What's reliable today that's on the Web, what is out of date information or misinformation, and what is the latest research and news on cooking oils or on any other nutraceutical or food product?

Don't write anything 'bad' about any commercial food product. Remember what happened to Oprah Winfrey when she discussed eating beef or hamburgers publicly on her show? She was sued by the beef industry. As a media professional, you can refer readers to medical journal articles or similar research. If a manufacturer or retailer loses money from what you wrote, you could be sued for damages. Instead, refer people to the published scientific research. A hot issue in the news currently is ethnicity and nutrition.

Food and Hispanic Populations

Do different ethnic groups have different or similar nutrition requirements for maximum health results? The article below on meeting the needs of the growing Hispanic population is reprinted here with the permission of the International Food Information Council. This article also appears online at: http://ific.org/foodinsight/2005/ja/hispoutreachfi405.cfm.

Adapting Outreach to Meet the Needs of the Growing Hispanic Population

Food Insight
July/August 2005

According to the Annual Demographic Supplement to the March 2002 Current Population Survey, the U.S. Census Bureau projects that the nation's Hispanic population will triple over the next half century. Nearly 67 million people of Hispanic origin will be added to the nation's population between 2000 and 2050. Their numbers are projected to grow from 35.6 million in 2000 to 102.6 million in 2050, an increase of 188 percent. Their share of the nation's population would nearly double, from 12.6 percent in 2000 to 24.4 percent in 2050.[1]

In addition, Census Bureau estimates show the Hispanic population in the United States has reached an all-time high of 38.8 million. The nation's Hispanic population grew much faster than the population as a whole, increasing from 35.6 million on April 1, 2000 to 38.8 million on July 1, 2002. This growth makes the Hispanic community the nation's largest minority community, representing 13.3% of the U.S. population.[2]

We can see results of this growth in the ever-increasing diversity and vibrancy of the towns and cities where we live and work and in the people we meet every day. To meet the information needs of this growing population a broader outreach to the entire Hispanic community is essential. There is a great need for all types of credible information including information on food safety, nutrition, and health.

With this in mind, the IFIC Foundation has joined the outreach effort by developing a Spanish-language Web site to provide sound, science-based information on food safety, nutrition and health to the Hispanic community within the United States, as well as for Spanish speakers around the world. The IFIC Foundation's Spanish-language Web site (http://ific.org/sp) provides a wealth of *free* information on everything from child and adolescent nutrition, to obesity and weight management, to food allergies and asthma, and everything in between.

In its report on the characteristics of the Hispanic population in the United States, the Census Bureau states that more than 1-in-3 Hispanics are under age 18, and that Hispanic children represent 18 percent of all children in the United

States.[2] Among the timely and relevant Spanish-language information you'll find on http://ific.org/sp for children and adolescents is a backgrounder on *Nutrition, Health & Physical Activity during Childhood and Early Adolescence*, as well as a poster for caregivers and parents on preventing childhood choking.

Accordingly, if more than 1-in-3 Hispanics is under age 18, then 2-in-3 Hispanics are over age 18. The IFIC Foundation has a wealth of credible, science-based information for this older segment of the population as well.

On http://ific.org/sp, you'll find a Spanish language poster for food service workers, addressing food allergies, as well as extensive Spanish-language documents on nutrition, health, and physical activity; functional foods; dietary fats and fat replacers; low-calorie sweeteners; fructose; food ingredients; pesticides and food safety; and mercury and fish. In addition, the IFIC Foundation's bi-monthly newsletter, *Food Insight* is posted on http://ific.org/sp.

New Spanish-language documents are uploaded regularly, and http://ific.org/sp users can sign up via e-mail to receive new and updated Spanish-language information as well as *Food Insight*.*

We encourage you to visit http://ific.org/sp and see for yourself!

[1] U.S. Census Bureau (http://www.census.gov/Press-Release/www/releases/archives/population/001720.html)

[2] U.S. Census Bureau (http://www.census.gov/PressRelease/www/releases/archives/hispanic_origin_population/001130.html)

*Please note, all e-mails from IFIC.org will be in English.

Related Information:

- IFIC.org en español

5

Nutrition Journalism Careers, Training, and Careers in Consumer Economics Communications

As a consumer communications writer or nutritionist in journalism, you have a problem to solve—clearing up public confusion due to overwhelming nutrition information in the news. Your bargaining tool is substance. You'll have to offer the oldest and largest media corporations substance over style when the major media increasingly is offering style over substance to promote branding and to sell American produce and products to the public. See the Web site titled, Journalism.org—Researches, Resources & Ideas to Improve Journalism at http://www.journalism.org/.

According to the "Overview" from Journalism.org's article titled "The State of News Media 2004," an Annual Report on American Journalism posted on the Web site at: http://www.stateofthenewsmedia.org/narrative_overview_eight.asp?media=1, an increasing number of news outlets are "chasing relatively static or even shrinking audiences for news." If audiences are shrinking for general mass media news, then the growth must be in ethnic, alternative, and online media. Do you break into the nutrition and consumer science alternate media, or compete for the few jobs at the top in the nutrition and consumer sections of the general mass media? It all depends on your expertise, training, and credibility in nutrition.

Writing about nutrition falls under alternative media and also may be applied to niche media such as online and ethnic food media. The major money is pouring into media dissemination, not in collecting news, such as compiling news clips or information in a "holding tank" or database. So you see news going out around the world more than you see companies collecting and storing information. The job of a news reporter, for example, is to collect news. That's not where the money is going.

Since newsrooms are cutting back in staff, to find a job in journalism, you need to have expertise—degrees—in some other field of concentration so you have a specialty. If you're a registered dietician with a Masters degree in nutrition/dietetics and have an undergraduate degree B.S. or A.S. in nursing (and licensed as a registered nurse) you have two professions to choose from before you take a few courses in journalism and writing to polish your ability to explain science in plain language to the public.

If this is your route, you may have an A.S. degree in registered nursing and be a licensed registered nurse from a community college. Then you finish your B.S. degree in nutrition or nutrition and nursing at a four-year university.

Finally, you finish a master's degree in dietetics and become a registered dietician with a specialty. Your elective courses in journalism and professional writing give you the professional expertise you need to begin as a journalist in nutrition and/or medical writing.

You can join a professional association such as the American Medical Writer's Association and take their continuing education seminars in medical writing. At this point, you have two niche specialties to help you break into journalism as a professional science writer with a nutrition or nutrition and nursing specialty. All you'd need are a few courses in journalism to learn how to write the news in short paragraphs and clear language.

Newspapers are not only cutting their staff. They also are cutting the time reporters have to gather the news and write tightly. If you don't have expertise in your area of specialty, the time-related pressure to gather news and write will be enormous. Read your own daily newspaper for quality. When you're writing about nutrition or health, the quality can't fail.

Cable news repeats itself without much updating. What you see on TV is "the end product" according to the article, "The State of the News Media 2004." Maybe you're seeing 24-hour media on TV, but how is the information ordered? Is it more chaotic than you'd read in print?

Do journalistic standards on TV or radio vary too much for the average consumer? Are people perceptive enough to notice? Yes, they are. What do they do with their perceptions that aren't perceived by radio talk show hosts as complaining by emotionally disturbed or angry callers?

Companies are interested in delivering mass audiences to the advertisers that support the media. News is sent across a variety of 'platforms.' Is news separated from advertising? Will news meet standards set by people audiences will never see? News delivery styles presented in the morning is different from news delivery styles presented in the evening.

Identity and brand become major issues because people who watch daytime TV are treated differently in content and attitude from those who watch prime time TV in the evening. The demographic of daytime TV viewers is different from the demographic of evening viewers.

Late night TV and early evening news TV contains shock advertising such as loud ambulance sirens and dramatizations of older people dying alone at home, addressed to mature adults living in fear of degenerative disease-related ailments or sudden illness. The ad agencies already know that older people turn on a certain type of animal, comedy, or travel TV show to make them laugh or see travel vistas because they can't sleep, possibly due to worry about their health. Shock advertising is used to sell electronic devices and drugs.

Before you choose a career in journalism, look at various media-related polls. These polls are online. Use the key word "media polls" in your Internet search engine. There are polls showing that the news media is driven by financial motives. General assignment reporters without professional expertise in one area such as science writing may have harder times finding jobs because of the downsizing of those who collect news. Polls emphasizing lack of professionalism in news are increasing. Consumers who read news want to see emphasis on public interest research.

As a nutrition writer, your focus is public interest research. The number of reporters employed by newspapers and magazines are decreasing. Shrinking space is the problem. The goal is to make room for more advertising and promotions. Prices charged to advertisers are going up, but advertising are being slapped with shrinking audiences. More costs are cut, and more audiences are lost.

Is the answer niche publishing? Convergence is the rule. Newspapers, magazines, and major book publishers are merging and/or converging. Online journalism is converging with older media, not replacing the old media and not creating new niches at increasing profits. So where are new niches being created if not by the old media now online?

Newspapers and major media TV are now in direct competition online. People want involvement and immediacy. In nutrition journalism you have individuals seeking to tailor their food to their genes, metabolism, and body type. All that's needed are professionals in nutrition who also are professionals in journalism.

If the profits that underwrite online newsgathering aren't there, will the World Wide Web decline as a news medium where now competing major media—the large TV stations and the largest daily newspapers—compete for decreasing audience participation? Debate this controversy. Use it for your term paper if you're still a student. If you're a writer or documentarian, write about it for a freelance submission to a publication. Produce a short documentary video or MP3 audio file for a Podcast or RSS syndication on a Web site.

If you are seeking a career in consumer communications, check the polls and economic results before you forecast where the profession of consumer communicator is headed. The major interview question is: "Who underwrites news gathering?" It's an economic issue, ripe for debate.

To debate consumer communications are a career, first you have to list and research who manipulates the press. Who buys consumer communications news and features? Next, you look at supply and demand. News outlets are increasing, especially in the ethnic, alternative, and specialty arena. As outlets increase, a seller's market for information is created due to competition.

News stories have too few sources, especially when related to health-related research findings. Reporters complain of the stress from too much work assigned to be completed in too few hours.

This pressure wears down the reporter's health. It's one of the reasons why so many journalists (with graduate degrees) leave time-pressured reporting careers to become community college journalism educators.

"Checkbook journalism" is created when TV reporters compete to be 'first' in obtaining interviews (scoops) with celebrities involved in the most current, controversial, and conspicuous news stories in order to increase their leverage over competing news stations.

For further information, read the 2004 study of the State of American Journalism, the Project for Excellence in Journalism, Columbia University Graduate School of Journalism, New York. Pew Charitable Trusts funded the study.

You live in an age where diverse content itself creates new markets. The media is indeed using a wider range of feature articles, especially related to health and food. The "new diversity" in the media emphasizes consumer communications, lifestyle, and entertainment, including food related to entertainment such as restaurant reviews (because they bring in advertising revenues).

Lighter fare is the name of the game in the media today. Presenting nutrition information as lighter fare is in demand. What it boils down to is scientific findings presented as easy-to-understand news written in plain language.

You have small publications for various ethnic audiences and you have the mass media featuring "lighter fare/consumer news." Branding takes up a huge portion of the media—promotions, teases, and commercials. Cooking shows on cable and satellite TV stations are increasing. Note the number of alternative health cooking shows, ethnic cooking, and cooking fast or competing chefs presented as entertainment.

Consumer communications professionals who write about diet, personal finance, and lifestyle should be pleased that diet, personal finance, and lifestyle features are replacing hard news in general interest publications and news magazines.

Newspapers, with all their downsizing of reporters, still employ more reporters than TV or radio. Magazines are overwhelmed with hundreds of freelance submissions and/or query letters. Web sites, similar to newspapers, are often set up by major newspapers, hire content producers, and compete for credibility and 'hits' against the individual news 'blog' or Web site with in-depth health or diet information referring readers to medical journal articles.

What types of magazine titles are increasing? Look for niche specialty publications ranging from alternative health topics, mountain biking, running, doll or toy collecting, to topics related to older adults. A nutritionist can write an article on food for a mountain biking publication.

Emphasize what portable food is best to carry when mountain biking and how certain foods affect the ability to bike for longer periods uphill. Or write on how biorhythms affect the body differently each hour of the day, or on topics related to stress and performance.

TV dominates international news. The Pew Research Center for the People and the Press reported in its 2003 study that "83% of Americans obtained most of their news information from TV, 42% from newspapers, 19% from radio, and 15% from the Internet."

Do these statistics reflect accuracy when more than one answer on survey questions was allowed? That's why research from a variety of sources is necessary before you make decisions. Specialized audiences reading high-quality content from publications with smaller circulations are where consumer communicators are more likely to find markets for what they write. Also look at public radio stations, and economics publications as possible markets for consumer communications.

The older media still has good profits. If you think the largest, oldest newspapers are going broke, think again. In 2003, these types of newspapers earned about a 20% profit. Local TV stations earned double that amount. Is there a relationship to that profit and the increasing number of cooking shows on satellite TV stations? Radio news represents only 11% of the revenues of the major radio corporations. You have health food stores sponsoring radio shows on nutrition that feature guests who are physicians, nutritionists, or nutrition book authors.

There are many paid infomercials on radio featuring vitamin manufacturing company representatives, some of whom have written books on alternative health. You have almost no cooking shows on radio, but numerous alternative health-oriented and body-mind-spirit types of radio programs. These shows draw a niche audience interested in the alternative health and nutrition product markets. Nutritionists who write books and articles can find a promotional market as guests on these types of radio shows as an alternative to paid infomercials.

The media today is fragmented. It's more difficult for advertisers to attract an audience. Spanish-language newspapers have increased seven fold in the decade 1990-2001 from $111 million to $786 million. For further information, The Latino Print Network contains the actual statistics.

If you're bilingual in Spanish and English, you might try to write for Spanish language newspapers published in the USA focusing on your particular area of consumer communications or nutrition. The Internet is still relying on the largest, oldest media. Time will tell what the profits will be.

In the meantime, the resources for gathering news is small and declining, whereas the outlets are spread thin as ice with small, lower-paying alternative and ethnic niche outlets increasing. The rich are getting richer. The big companies are growing larger. What the richest companies want is to have everything under one roof.

Those who write the news and features want diversity of points of view. Magazine consolidation is a bit slower than that of the other media. The largest magazine corporations include Time Warner, Hearst, Advance, and Primedia. There actually are at least 25 large media firms.

You could apply to these largest firms to intern as a nutrition or consumer communications writer, food photography stylist, or public relations professional.

Newspapers have lost about 2,200 professional employees during the decade of 1990-2001. If you want to see actual numbers and resources since 2001, consult the changing statistics published by the American Society of Newspaper Editors. There are fewer newspapers today than there were a decade ago.

In the past, printers typeset newspaper stories. Today, the growing amount of production work is done on computers in the newsroom rather than by composing room workers, linotype setters, or printers. Computers helped to reduce the mechanical work of the composing room.

Communications is moving toward digital media. For nutritionists who write, the choice is whether to write about the effects on the human body of homogenized milk or the much cheaper homogenized content relying on news wires, podcasts, and RSS feeds. Technology is replacing newsgathering skills because it costs less.

Then why be a nutritionist who writes for the mass media? You write in order to distinguish yourself as an expert offering substance with style. There's competition between style and substance in the media. As a nutritionist who writes, you are able to attract a growing audience.

How you compete is by offering content that is less similar to what's currently in the news. The major media competes by offering similar content. Everything looks too much alike in the daily news and in major magazines. That's why audiences are declining. The more the larger media compete, the more crowded the space grows in which the largest, oldest media operates. With so little space to maneuver, the media turns to branding as a solution.

As the largest media outlets emphasize more branding, the nutrition writer offers results and solves the problem of attracting more audience by offering diverse styles with more substance. Who has the most diverse style and the most substance today? It's offering food and alternative health as entertainment—as long as you have the medical journal articles references to back up your word with proven, credible studies and research. Physicians most popular in the media have long known this.

Too often, the public think of journalists who write about nutrition as not being adequately trained. Read some of the studies published by the American Society of Newspaper Editors. People still think that journalists sensationalize the news in order to advance their jobs and sell newspapers. As a professional in the nutrition field, consumer science, or medical writing, you need to show you are a moral, professional who cares enough about your reader's health to reveal your resources in credible, medical studies and journals.

What Can You Expect from a Career in Consumer Communications?

The days are not over when you might end up typing other people's ideas or teaching high school (pretty good pay if you get tenure and then advance to principal), unless you become an expert and a generalist. Getting a PhD is one way to become an expert in a specific subject. With a Masters degree, you're competing against too many other people with Master's degrees in communications.

There's another way—get a degree in an area so specialized that you can use your general and specialized skills at the same time. To overcome expenses, look for paid externships and internships, especially with the government, health care industry, or with the media in industries most likely to offer you a job.

Stay away from the downsizing, merging arms of the media. Consumer journalism is expanding with niche publications, investigative businesses, and a few, specialized, new government agencies. Journalism careers emphasizing nutrition issues and controversies may concentrate in ten directions:

1. consumer journalism

2. food journalism emphasizing recipes and features about regional or ethnic foods for the food section of newspapers and magazines

3. cooking shows on TV

4. restaurant critiquing/reviews for newspapers and magazines

5. health, fitness, and alternative medicine

6. medical writing

7. body, mind, spirit

8. travel writing focusing on food

9. writing about wine and viticulture for trade journals, newspapers, or consumer magazines

10. home economics journalism (family and consumer sciences)

To train for any of these concentrations, there are professional associations, majors at universities on the undergraduate or graduate level, and seminars for continuing education sponsored by trade and professional associations or universities. Decide first whether your concentration is to be in nutrition or in journalism, or divided equally as far as training and writing.

Training for a career in Family and Consumer Communications

If you want to write cookbooks, do you train in journalism, consumer sciences, or in cooking? Where and how do you train for a career in consumer communications? Food writing and agricultural writing lead to diverse careers in consumer education communications. Before the 1960s, agricultural journalism had been the major of choice for people who wanted to write about nutrition, food, ethnobotany, and special diets for the general consumer, mass media, advertising or public relations agencies, agricultural trade journals, wires and syndicated services, or scientific publications.

Majors in agricultural journalism were offered at universities located mostly in agricultural areas. Urban universities offered courses in dietetics, home economics, or nutrition and foods. The ethnobotany students usually majored in botany or plant genetics.

Today, agricultural journalism is still a career that attracts students interested in farming or agricultural sciences. It's a major students may choose as an alternative to a major in dietetics with a minor in journalism. There also are actual university majors and degree programs on undergraduate or graduate levels where you can train specifically in the field of nutrition communications. Alternatives include medical journalism for those who have majored in one of the life sciences such as ethnobotany. For more information, you can research the American Medical Writer's Association. The association's Web site is at: http:// www.amwa.org/.

If you're more interested in agricultural journalism than in writing about health, pharmaceuticals, genetics, and medicine, research a group known as the North American Agricultural Journalists. According to its Web site at: http:// naaj.tamu.edu/, the North American Agricultural Journalists "is a professional, international group of agricultural editors and writers with a membership spanning the United States and Canada." Formerly the Newspaper Farm Editors of America, and then the National Association of Agricultural Journalists, it was organized in 1952 to promote the highest ideals of journalism and agricultural coverage.

"Eligible for memberships are journalists in North America that report or edit agricultural news for newspapers, magazines, wires and syndicated services and are independent of agricultural organizations and businesses. Members who retire or resign from their journalism positions may become associate members. Students interested in a career in agricultural writing also are encouraged to join."

Home Economics Journalism Changes Its Name to Consumer Economics Communications

In the 1960s, when an increasing number of male journalists began to take an interest in consumer economics communications, many wished the home economics journalism major would have a more neutral-sounding label such as "consumer communications." The home economics major drew interest mostly from women, although men interested in the housing industry usually selected a major in residential real estate.

Pre-medical students interested in nutrition careers often would major in one of the life sciences. For those who went on to medical school, the lack of nutrition courses soon became evident to patients asking their doctors questions about diets. Physicians usually had only few hours of training in nutrition and would refer patients to registered dieticians that had degrees in dietetics and nutrition. The mass media often assigned reporters with little or no training in nutrition and the life sciences to write articles for the food page, which were limited to recipes and restaurant reviews. The agricultural trade journal thrived, but interested farming communities and industries.

Fifty years ago most women reporters were delegated to the "women's page" that largely hosted food, society, and lifestyle features. By the end of the 1960s, health lifestyles, parenting, and nutrition-related articles began to replace the home-economics oriented 'women's' pages with articles or tips on health care, home repair, restaurant reviews, food information, shopping, and taste. The 'women's pages weren't for only women anymore, but began to focus more on self-help, health, exercise, food quality, society, lifestyles, and even entertainment.

Not many male journalism students interested in writing for consumer publications chose a major with a name such as "home economics journalism." They chose alternative communications majors such as "advertising" and took minors in business, various life sciences, or financial economics. Some students did become registered dieticians by taking a major in nutrition.

Other students obtained graduate degrees in journalism, but this was costly for those who had to find jobs right out of college. Also graduate degrees in nutrition were more in demand than graduate degrees in communications. Those who had PhDs in nutrition with minors in journalism had choice jobs as the experts that other journalists interviewed.

Some worked in industrial kitchens for food manufacturers as product developers and testers. Others became cooking show hosts or book authors. However, most popular cook book writers don't have doctorates in nutrition research. Others own famous restaurants, are executive chefs, or TV personalities.

Numerous students interested in the marriage of nutrition and journalism went into careers in copywriting, public relations, food testing, food styling for ad photographers, or special diet supervision careers in hospital environments. Others entered careers in news writing and consumer science publishing.

Nutrition journalism also is known at different universities under different names for the undergraduate or graduate major. What used to be called Home Economics journalism is now called Consumer and Family Communications at some schools and nutrition/dietetics journalism at other schools.

According to the University of Wisconsin-Madison's Family and Consumer Communications Web site describing Family and Consumer Communications as a university major (and the major's history) at: http://www.sohe.wisc.edu/depts/history/depts/fcc.htm, (formerly Family and Consumer Journalism; formerly Home Economics Journalism), numerous students prepared for journalism careers by obtaining a degree in agricultural journalism. In decades past, journalists prepared for their careers by majoring in many different fields.

According to the University of Wisconsin-Madison's Family and Consumer Communications Web site at: http://www.sohe.wisc.edu/depts/history/depts/fcc.htm, (reprinted with permission) "Even before the introduction of a major in Home Economics Journalism in 1933, some students had prepared for careers in journalism by completing majors in other fields of home economics and taking electives in the Journalism or Agricultural Journalism Department. Among these early graduates was Nell Nichols, who earned a Masters in foods and nutrition with a minor in Journalism in 1917, and who went to write for and later edit *Women's Home Companion*, in addition to authoring numerous cookbooks.

"During the early decades of the Home Economics Journalism major, students could choose to enrich their formal studies by writing for the <u>*Wisconsin Country Magazine*</u>, the student newspaper of the College of Agriculture. Students also gained experience in broadcasting by appearing on the WHA program Homemakers' Program under <u>Aline Hazard</u>'s supervision. There they might present a talk on interior decorating, on better buying, or on how to plan a buffet supper.

"Between 1951 and 1974, the Home Economics Journalism major was included in the <u>Home Economics Education and Extension</u> Department. In 1974, with the introduction of the Home Economics Communications (later renamed Family and Consumer Communication) Department, the major finally achieved a greater degree of prominence. In addition to teaching students to employ an ever-expanding range of communication technologies, faculty members and students within the department have conducted research on the ways in which families and consumers use and respond to these media."

The Business Journalism Route to Consumer Economics Communications Careers

Another path to writing or public speaking careers in consumer economics communications leads to a major in business or economics journalism. For example, the business journalism program at Washington and Lee University, Lexington, VA, bridges two historic strengths of the university: its journalism department and its undergraduate School of Commerce, Economics and Politics. The program also taps the resources at the Washington and Lee School of Law.

One way into a journalism career is by graduating from law school and then concentrating on writing about law as it relates to food and related topics. Another way is to take an undergraduate degree in food science with a minor in journalism and then go to law school specializing in agricultural or food law. Another route is to study for an undergraduate degree in Science and Environmental Writing. Such a degree is offered by Lehigh University's Department of Journalism & Communication. Details are at the University's Web site at: http://www.lehigh.edu/~injrl/sciwrit/.

Whatever path you choose, an internship is the way to get experience while you're still in school. Some journalists take a major in broadcasting and a minor in home economics or consumer sciences. Others take a double major in agricultural journalism and agriculture.

Choose your main field of concentration or interest, and then build the writing skills around your expertise in one area. You need to be both a generalist and a specialist to find the right job or best-fit internship.

Maybe you like travel or geography and want to work or intern with the Foreign Development Division of the U.S. Department of Agriculture. You can begin by researching what types of work that division does. At the least, you can develop a feature article for a publication on the subject.

6

How Journalists Understand and Interpret Food and Health-Related Scientific Studies

Food misinformation, the childhood obesity and diabetes epidemics, and the proliferation of fad diets are important issues in nutrition today, ripe for debate, discussion, and investigative reporting. An equally important topic for discussion, debate, or media coverage is: who controls the quality of nutritional supplements and what health benefits have been proven scientifically?

There's a book titled, *Encyclopedia of Diet Fads* (Hardcover) by Marjolijn Bijlefeld, Sharon K. Zoumbaris. Greenwood Press, 2003. It covers fad diets of the past and current times. *Encyclopedia of Diet Fads* emphasizes weight loss problems aimed at young people. It's an excellent resource when you want to compare patterns and fads in diets to the current child and adolescent obesity epidemic.

What nutrition journalists also need to publish is an encyclopedia written in plain language that organizes current nutrition research/studies proven not to be flawed. Such a guide would show what health benefits certain foods and nutritional supplements offer to the general public.

It would clearly explain why the products should not be taken by people taking certain medicines or combinations of medicines, or why the products or foods should not be taken by those with certain conditions. Consumers need an encyclopedia backed up by credible studies for fact checking. Confused readers are looking for current nutrition research that discusses the health benefits of food, supplements, and lifestyles.

Who would write this type of guide? If most physicians receive only a few hours of training in nutrition in medical school, would the work require a team of biochemists, registered dieticians, physicians, and geneticists? Should the publisher also include a nutrition journalist to organize the words—group them under similar topics, and make sure such a guide was written at the fifth grade reading level of daily newspapers?

Nutrition and consumer communicators need to include the pros and cons of using herbs or other food products. When writing about herbs, a nutrition journalist needs to include when not to use them. Not all herbs are meant for all people. One example would be the herb, rosemary. It's a powerful stimulant that should be avoided by those with heart or seizure problems. Yet there are few warnings when rosemary is added to food products, oils, or vitamins as a preservative. This type of nutrition information needs to reach the public, written in language that requires no science training.

There are herbs and plants that may stimulate the nervous system to possibly cause panic attacks in people with autonomic nervous system defects or those genetically at risk for anxiety or seizures. Those herbs and plants need warning on labels on products containing those herbs, extracts, acids, milk derivatives, or some other 'natural' plant products. Some food jars are labeled 'spices.' However, an ingredient such as MSG, which some are sensitive to, could also be labeled as a spice. The actual names of the spices should be present on food product labels, but many products only list the generic term 'spices.'

There are few articles widely disseminated to the public warning about reactions to products for those with panic disorder or "the anxiety gene." Everyone knows about peanut allergies, but who writes about the effects of herbs such as rosemary, or caffeine, and other plants or even plant-based aphrodisiacs that may stimulate panic attacks in those with "the anxiety gene?" The studies still lie in the medical journals, largely unread by the public.

Holding the Public's Attention

How do you hold the public's attention when they already are confused by too much and too technical information and food publicity? According to the article reprinted below, with permission of the International Food Information Council, getting the reader's attention in a startling headline is one hook, but keeping the public's attention requires explaining clearly what supporting studies accurately report. The article, originally published by IFIC Review in September 2001, addresses even today the problem of confusion caused by the overwhelming flood of health information published in the media. (Also see the article posted by IFIC at http://ific.org/publications/reviews/scientificir.cfm?renderforprint=1.

IFIC Review: How to Understand and Interpret Food and Health-Related Scientific Studies

---

Source: http://ific.org © 2005 International Food Information Council Foundation

September 2001

Kumquats Found to Prevent Cancer! *Exercise + eggplant = longer life!!*

Obviously, these "headlines" are fictitious, but they got your attention, didn't they? Reports of new research findings in the area of food and health grab the attention of Americans from all walks of life. After all, food and health are central concerns to each of us. Reporters, professors, and health professionals all want the latest information—as do consumers. A single study and the reports surrounding it can send crowds of people in search of the latest food or supplement that holds promise for good health. Remember how virtually any food containing oats or oat bran practically flew off supermarket shelves in 1990 after an oat bran-cholesterol study was publicized?

Frustrated and confused by the tremendous amount of food and health information being communicated today, Americans look for simple certainties to help them protect their health through diet. The trouble is that single studies rarely provide such certainty, although they often make for great headlines.

The media, health professionals, and educators are the gatekeepers of today's food and health information. They determine, for the most part, what consumers hear, read, and believe about food and health. Along with that comes the responsibility to provide the facts, put them in perspective, and help people determine how the findings may affect their behavior and lives. Fulfilling this responsibility requires that new studies be critically reviewed before being publicized. News releases and study abstracts, although helpful for "previewing" research, do not provide the information necessary to accurately and responsibly report findings to the public.

Happily, with practice, the process of critically reviewing scientific research becomes easier and less time-consuming. This *IFIC Review* is designed to help members of the media, health professionals, and educators understand how to read and evaluate food and health-related scientific studies. It presents an overview of key information to look for, questions to ask, and other important considerations.

A Process of Discovery and Debate

To consumers, it often seems that contradictory studies about food and health appear in the media almost weekly, leaving many to wonder why researchers can't get it right the first time. The answer is not an easy one to swallow, because to accept it means we must accept uncertainty.

The scientific process is a road of discovery. It is a process of gaining knowledge about the universe through the observation of measurable evidence (1). Contrary to what many people may believe, this "road" is not necessarily a straight one. That is, researchers may take different directions of exploration, causing the "road" to twist, turn, and sometimes even backtrack or come to a dead end before the facts are uncovered. Even then the facts may be only part of a larger, partially understood phenomenon, which requires that more research be conducted before we find the answers.

As a result, the scientific process—how studies are designed, conducted, and reported—frequently generates a great deal of debate. Tracking the debate is often key to putting new research into context. With that in mind, new research studies published in scientific journals should be viewed as discussions among scientists. In these discussions, almost no one gets to have the final word, as it is rare that a study provides a final, complete answer (2). In fact, occasionally even old, accepted research results are revisited and discussed again. With the benefit of new information or technology, scientists sometimes see old results in a new light. The publication of research findings allows researchers to obtain input on their work, which not only confirms or contradicts their results but also adds to the body of literature on a subject and helps shape future research.

The bottom line is that dialogues characterized by cycles of revisions, conjectures, assertions, and contradictions are frequently key to investigating a subject. In addition, although such cycles often frustrate nonscientists and can contribute to increasing public skepticism about advice on food and health, it is important to understand that science is evolutionary, not revolutionary (3). Because scientific research explores the unknown, uncertainty is an unavoidable part of current investigations. Only through repeated research and analyses do certainties emerge.

Types of Research Studies: What They Are & When They Are Used

Broadly, research can be divided into two categories: observational and experimental. Within these categories, there are three basic methods by which scientists investigate questions about food and health (4). It is essential to understand what each method can and cannot do.

Observational Research

Observational research involves examination of specific factors in defined groups of subjects to investigate the relationships between those factors and aspects of health or illness (5). For example, an observational study may focus on the body weight of healthy women aged 50 or older and its relationship to blood pressure in that group. Observational research can only suggest relationships, however. It takes experimental research to determine cause and effect.

Epidemiological research is often observational, but it may also be experimental. It is the study of the distribution and determinants of diseases or other health outcomes in human populations (6). It seeks to expose potential associations between aspects of health (such as cancer and heart disease) and diet, lifestyle, habits, or other factors within populations.

Although epidemiological studies are useful for *suggesting* relationships between two factors, it is important to remember the basic limitation of epidemiological studies: they do not necessarily indicate cause and effect (5). In fact, the associations that they indicate can actually turn out to be coincidental. A simple example of this would be a study which suggested that driving a Cadillac was associated with increased risk for cardiovascular disease. In this case, the fact that the car was a Cadillac was a coincidence. The association revealed by the study should have been between driver characteristics (gender, age, weight) and the disease.

Observational epidemiological research may be most revealing when considered in the context of what experimental research suggests about a subject (7). For example, to assess whether an association discovered in an epidemiological study is real and not the result of bias or confounding factors, researchers may conduct a randomized clinical trial to confirm a suspected cause-and-effect relationship.

Experimental Research

In experimental research, study subjects (whether human or animal) are selected according to relevant characteristics and are then randomly assigned to either an experimental group or a control group (5). Random assignment ensures that factors (known as *variables*) that may affect the outcome of the study are distributed equally among the groups and therefore could not lead to differences in the effect of a treatment. The experimental group(s) is then given a treatment (sometimes called an *intervention*), and the results are compared with those for the control group, which does not receive a treatment (or which receives a placebo, or fake treatment). Any differences in results between the groups can then be attributed to the treatment; that is, the effect can be considered to be caused by the treatment. Controlled experimental research can be fraught with errors, easily becoming uncontrolled. Sometimes these flaws are easily spotted, but in many cases it is worth asking experts—they know what to look for.

Basic research generates data by investigating biochemical substances or biological processes (4). It is often undertaken to confirm observations or discover how a particular process works. For example, an experiment might take place to examine how vitamin E may help prevent oxidation of LDL (low-density lipoprotein) cholesterol, a process believed to play a role in the development of heart disease. This basic research is just part of a larger effort to understand how diet can help reduce risk for heart disease.

Basic research may be conducted in vitro (such as in test tubes) or with animals. Research with animals is an important tool in determining how humans may react when exposed to particular substances. However, it is important to note that, due to differences in physiology and the fact that animals are routinely exposed to levels of compounds far higher than those that human populations typically encounter, one cannot assume that results from studies with animals can be generalized to humans.

Clinical trials deal with the experimental study of human subjects. Trials may attempt to determine whether the findings of basic research are applicable to humans or to confirm the results of epidemiological research. Studies may be small, with a limited number of participants, or they may be large intervention trials that seek to discover the outcome of treatments on entire populations. "Gold standard" clinical trials are double-blind placebo-controlled studies that use random assignment of subjects to experimental and control groups.

Talking with the Experts

Journalists, educators, and health professionals who need to quickly distill the findings of a new study should consider contacting the study authors or other scientists familiar with the body of research on the topic. Experts can answer questions and provide insight that both novice and experienced readers may not be able to unearth by themselves. In addition, interviewing scientists other than the study author can bring valuable insights and contribute to a more balanced perspective of the study.

Questions you may want to ask a study's author or other experts include the following:

- *Could the study be interpreted to say something else?*

  Scientists often reach different conclusions from the same or similar data, so asking "What's your take on this study" is not unusual. The rationale for different conclusions may be important when putting a study's findings into context.

- *Are there any methodological flaws in the study that should be considered when making conclusions?*

  The more experts who review a study, the more likely potential flaws—such as confounding variables—will be discovered.

- *Are the study's results generalizable to other groups?*

  Consumers want to know how research affects them. If study results are applicable only to a narrow group of people, it should be reported as such.

- *How does this work fit with the body of research on the subject?*

  Even a well-written article may not include a discussion of all relevant research because of space limitations. Yet, it is extremely important to know—and communicate to consumers—whether a study is confirming previous research and therefore adding more weight to scientific beliefs or whether the study's results and conclusions make a wild departure from current thinking on the subject.

What to Look for When Critically Reviewing Scientific Studies

To enhance communication among scientists and to facilitate replication of the study, published research generally follows an established format. This section of this *Review* highlights important information to look for and questions to ask yourself or to pose to experts. This information should help you to understand each part of the study. Be aware that exactly where the information appears in different articles varies somewhat.

Abstract

The abstract of a published study serves to briefly answer the basic questions about what was studied, how it was done, and the results. Its primary purpose is to allow readers to make an initial evaluation of whether a study is of interest without having to read the complete paper. If only we could just peruse the abstract and consider our review of the study complete! Unfortunately, that is not the case. Abstracts do not provide nearly enough detail to enable readers to assess the validity of a study or put it into context. These can be done only by thoroughly reviewing the rest of the study.

What is a Double-Blind Placebo-Controlled Study? (sidebar)

Considered the "gold standard" of clinical research studies, the double-blind placebo-controlled study provides dependable findings that are free of bias introduced by either the subject or the researcher.

In this type of study, neither the subject nor the researcher conducting the study knows whether the test substance or a placebo has been administered. For the results to be valid and to ensure that the subject cannot violate the "blindness," the placebo and the test substance must be virtually identical (i.e., look, smell, and taste similar).

The "blindness" of the study is crucial. It eliminates the possibility that a participant's personal beliefs will undermine the study's validity. It also prevents the researcher's expectations from influencing the test results.

Introduction

The introduction section "welcomes" the reader to the study. It eases the reader into the research by presenting the question that the researcher seeks to answer or the problem or hypothesis that the study addresses (8). It explains *why* the study will be conducted, which gives the reader a clue to the potential importance of the research. It also expands a little more on *how* the research will be conducted. The introduction can be divided into two major parts: the Background section and the Purpose section.

Background: The background information presented in the introduction of a study tells why the researchers think the study is important (8). It should reflect a comprehensive knowledge of the body of research on the subject and should brief the reader on both the previous studies that support the concepts or theories of the current study and those that do not. In essence, it brings the reader up to speed on current thinking and presents the researcher's rationale for pursuing the study.

Purpose: The stated purpose essentially defines the study (9). It dictates how a study will be conducted: the research design, the variables that will be measured, how information will be collected and analyzed, and what conclusions may be drawn.

In some instances you may find that the study does not seem to be appropriately designed or conducted to achieve its purpose. For example, the type of study may not yield the type of information required to answer the stated question or the study population may not fit the purpose. Consultation of experts about these points can be very helpful in determining the validity of the study's conclusions.

Key Questions to Ask:

- *What are the inherent limitations of this type of study?*
- *Does the research design fit the stated purpose of the study?*
- *Has the author omitted from the Background section important points that could have a meaningful effect on the study design or interpretation of the results?*

Methodology

The key question of the methodology section is "How?" This section should enable critical readers to determine whether the research is valid; that is, was it adequately designed to achieve its purpose (9)? Hence, the methodology section warrants careful review. It explains how the research was conducted and should give information in enough detail for the reader to evaluate the study. It should also enable the reader to understand to whom or what the study results apply. Important information featured in the methodology section includes the following (10):

- the setting of a study (in a clinic, laboratory, population, etc.)

- how variables were controlled (how did they adjust for specific subject qualities or outside influences that could affect the results?)

- the sample size

- the number of study groups

- the treatment or variables being observed (e.g., a vitamin supplement or specific diets)

- the length of the study

- how the data were collected

- how and by what statistical procedures the data were analyzed

The methodology section also provides information about the sampling method and whether subjects were randomly assigned or not (in experimental studies). Pay specific attention to these points, because they are among the first steps in conducting research, and flaws present here can render the results invalid.

Randomness in Selection and Assignment: The term "random sample" is familiar to most everyone, but exactly how subjects (the "sample") are selected for the study is of crucial importance. Among other things, the sampling method affects to whom the study results may be relevant.

If the subjects are selected randomly, that is, via a procedure in which all individuals in a population being studied have an equal chance of being selected, then the study results may be generalizable to that population (9). True random selection may be done using a table of random numbers generated by a computer. Calling people picked randomly out of a telephone book between the hours of 1:00 and 3:00 p.m. in the afternoon is not random sampling of the entire population of the United States, for instance. We can all think of a number of reasons why this is not truly random: some people don't have telephones, and some people have unlisted phone numbers. In addition, the sample would likely be light on full-time workers and would be weighted heavily with stay-at-home mothers, elderly and unemployed people, students, people who are ill, and people who work the night shift, for example.

The term "random" also applies to the assignment or the division of subjects into groups. Random assignment ensures that all subjects have an equal chance of being in the experimental and control groups and increases the probability that any unidentified variable will systematically occur in both groups with the same frequency.

Randomization is crucial to controlling for variables that researchers may not be aware of or cannot adequately control but that could affect the outcome of an experimental study (9). To determine the true effect of a treatment, researchers must carefully control for all variables that could affect the outcome of a study. Some of the variables are obvious, such as age, body weight, and gender.

To control for these differences, researchers match subjects in experimental and control groups so that they have similar characteristics. Some variables, such as heredity, are more difficult to control for. Still others may be unknown—because knowledge of human biology is still developing, for example. By randomly assigning subjects to study groups, the influence of such variables is minimized and any differences in results between groups can be attributed to the treatment.

A Question of Size—Sample Size, That Is: As you probably know from experience, the primary question about sample size is "Was it big enough to find an effect?" The answer is not always as easy to come by. In fact, it is often a matter of judgment.

For example, when studying the effect of a weight-loss drug, a researcher may decide that a sample size of 100 people is adequate because the effect is easily noted: How many pounds did those who received the drug lose, compared with those who did not receive the drug? However, when assessing the average fruit and vegetable consumption among children who participated in a school-based intervention program, several thousand children may be deemed necessary because the increase from such an intervention is likely to be relatively small.

That is, the diets of the children in experimental and control groups may not differ much in terms of fruit and vegetable intake, and therefore, the effect of the intervention might not be noticed. It is easier to spot a small effect when you are looking at results for a large sample.

A small sample size, however, does not necessarily mean that the study is flawed. For example, prospective clinical nutrition studies usually have just a small number of subjects because there are so many variables that need to be controlled. When reading a study, be sure to look for the rationale that the researcher used to decide the sample size.

Of Abstracts and News Releases (sidebar)

When deadlines loom near, it may be tempting to rely only on an abstract and a news release for information about a research study instead of taking time to examine the original published study. Resist the temptation! Abstracts and releases are not substitutes for original research. They simply do not provide enough information that can be used to judge the merits of a study or to accurately report the study results.

Medical journals, organizations, and universities regularly issue news releases to stimulate media coverage of research or conferences.

Make news releases and abstracts work for you by using them for ideas, story angles, quotes, potential interview subjects, and a "quick-and-dirty" overview of the research. Once you have a little background on the study, you can thoroughly review the original research article without spending too much additional time. Keep the "Key Questions to Ask" in mind as you review the article, and note specific questions that you have for experts as you go along.

A Word About Methodological Limitations: Often, limitations are placed on researchers—such as finances or the ethics of human testing—and these can severely restrict progress on the study and study results. Aside from these external limitations, there can also be internal limitations, such as those experienced when the current state of knowledge in a field (particularly as it relates to data collection instruments) is known to be limited. Any type of constraint—if it could affect the results of the study—should be openly discussed in the methodology or discussion sections of the study.

Key Questions to Ask:

- *Are there any major design flaws in this study?*
- *Are the data collection measures appropriate to answer the study questions?*
- *Were methodological limitations acknowledged and discussed?*
- *What influence might these limitations have had on the results?*

Results

Nobody will deny that reading a scientific study up to this point can be difficult and tedious. Now, however, we finally get to the really interesting stuff—the answers. The results section of a study does indeed provide what we might call answers but what scientists would call "data" and the statistical analyses of the data (8). For more precise communication, statistical measures are frequently used to convey the existence and strength of relationships.

The field of statistics is based on the quantification of information. Descriptive statistics present the information in an organized fashion so that it is easier to interpret (9). Some of the more familiar descriptive statistics include percentage, frequency, mean, and standard deviation. Descriptive statistics, however, do not provide information about cause and effect—this is the realm of inferential statistics. As the name implies, inferential statistics often involve making inferences from the results for the sample studied and extrapolating them to a larger population (8).

Understanding Statistical Significance: Without getting too technical, this brief discussion of significance will help the reader understand this common statistical measure.

Researchers generally calculate statistical significance and report it as a "*P* value." A *P* value is the probability of obtaining an effect or association in a study sample as or more extreme than the one observed if there was actually no effect in the population. If the results of a study are statistically significant, then the study may have indeed hit upon some real association or effect. The study author will identify what *P* value he or she has used in the analysis. A *P* value of less than 5 percent ($P < 0.05$) is fairly common and would be considered statistically significant (8). This means that the result would occur less than 5 percent of the time if there were no effect. More stringent levels of significance are $P < 0.01$ and $P < 0.001$.

If the results of a study are *not* statistically significant, the author may discuss the statistical power of the study. An in-depth discussion of power is beyond the scope of this *Review*; however, when present, information about statistical power in a study will help the reader understand whether the study had a chance of finding the answer to the research questions in the first place.

It is easy to get wrapped up in discussions of statistical significance when reading research, but it is important to remember that a statistically significant result does not necessarily mean that the results are important—or relevant to the public. In addition, a statistically significant finding does not guarantee that the research is without biases or confounding factors that could make the statistical value irrelevant (7). Statistical significance is only part of the picture; to get the whole picture, one must consider the context of the study—what other research on the subject reveals.

Communicating Risk: Attention readers: You "risk" misunderstanding and miscommunicating the results of the study if you do not fully comprehend the differences between relative and absolute risk.

Absolute risk refers to the actual risk of an occurrence—the chance that a specific outcome will occur. *Relative risk* puts risk in comparative terms—the outcome rate for people exposed to the factor in question compared with the outcome rate for those not exposed to the factor. A relative risk of >1 indicates an increased risk of the outcome under investigation; one of <1 indicates a decreased risk of the outcome. Relative risks are the most commonly used measure of morbidity or mortality in the medical literature today. However, in many cases the absolute risk is a far more relevant statistic for the public (11).

For example, suppose that a study shows that a man who brushes his teeth only once a day is 50 percent more likely to have all his teeth fall out in the next 10 years than others who brush their teeth twice per day. This is the relative risk. Yet, the absolute risk that all of the man's teeth will fall out may be only 1 percent. In this case, the relative risk makes the problem—a rare one anyway—seem more important than it really is. However, relative risk can also make a problem appear to be less important than it actually is. Therefore, it is important to consider both relative risk and absolute risk when discussing study results.

Key Questions to Ask:

- *What is the real and statistical significance of these results?*
- *To whom do these results apply?*
- *How do these results compare to those of other studies on the subject?*

Discussion

The discussion section of a study gives the reader some insight into the study subject area and often sheds new light on the results and their meaning. Alternative explanations for the results and the implications of the research may also be presented.

One of the most frequent errors in scientific research is drawing conclusions that are not adequately supported by the data. This may occur for a number of reasons: collection of insufficient or inadequate data, overgeneralization of results, methodological problems, or inherent limitations of the study design. This is why it is important to review the methodology section.

Sometimes, researchers stray from the scientific method by reporting conclusions that are unrelated to the research question that was tested. Although conclusions made in this manner may have merit, it is important to take a second look at whether the study was adequately designed and conducted to support the secondary conclusions (12).

Finally, be wary of absolute conclusions that profess to be the final word on a subject. Good research answers some questions and raises others. A call for more research to investigate particular issues that remain unclear or to replicate the current study findings frequently concludes a journal article.

Key Questions to Ask:

- *Are the conclusions supported by the data?*
- *Are the conclusions of the study related to the stated purpose of the study? If not, do the study design and results support the secondary conclusions?*

References

Experts in the subject area can usually tell rather quickly if key research has been omitted from the reference list. If this is the case, the researchers may have failed to adequately review, consider, and evaluate prior work in the field that could have benefited their current study. Also, a reference list that includes both older and newer relevant research can reassure the reader that the author has thoroughly reviewed the entire body of research for background and has not just considered the last few or first few studies conducted on the topic.

Also Consider...

Other issues that merit attention in the critical review of studies include the funding sources of a study and the appropriate use of editorials and letters to the editor.

Funding Source: Often, one hears a study being criticized—or its findings dismissed entirely—because it was funded by industry or another interested party. Many scientific journals today require that potential conflicts of interest be disclosed and sources of funding be referenced at the end of a paper. Although it is interesting to note the funding source of a study, it is unfair—and perhaps short-sighted—to simply negate the results solely on the basis of the funding source.

The reason that studies are often funded by organizations that may benefit from the results is obvious. After all, who else but an interested party would allocate the large amounts of money that good research often requires? For example, when a company is seeking approval for a new food ingredient, it is required by law to support adequate studies to demonstrate the ingredient's safety. The government—taxpayers—certainly would not invest millions of dollars to study food ingredients or products that may never come to market!

Ethical researchers do not manipulate data or design studies to support the funder's interests. Indeed, most members of industry do not want a "tell them what they want to hear" researcher; they want to know the real answers to their questions. A critical evaluation of research on its own merit is the best way to assess its validity and importance. If the study is good, its results will stand on their own—regardless of who supported the research.

Editorials and Letters-to-the-Editor: Editorials—or written opinions by experts in a field other than the authors of a study that the editorial addresses—may be one of the most valuable ways for readers to understand a study, its meaning, and its practical implications (13). Editorials often provide perspective on a study, discussing it in the context of other research, as well as identifying potential flaws that may affect the applicability or even veracity of the study results.

Although letters to the editor usually appear in issues following that in which a study is published, if a reader has the time to wait, such letters can be very useful to help identify potential problems with a study. At the least, they can be used as a continuing education tool on what to look for when critically reviewing studies.

Study results that are reported via letters to the editor, however, should not be taken at face value. They cannot substitute for peer-reviewed articles that provide the details necessary for readers to critically review the research.

Meet the Meta-Analysis (sidebar)

A meta-analysis is a statistical method of combining results from separate studies to derive overall conclusions about a question or hypothesis (14). Meta-analyses are conducted in an attempt to reconcile differences among studies in terms of their statistical power or sample sizes or to aggregate relevant findings across studies.

The procedure is most appropriate when examining studies that look at the same question and use similar methods to measure relevant variables. For example, using one type of meta-analysis, scientists examined the relationship between weight reduction and blood lipid levels (15). Although individual studies showed inconsistent results, pooling of data from 70 similar studies showed significant decreases in the levels of total cholesterol and other blood lipids due to weight loss.

The technique of meta-analysis is not without limitations, however. Data from flawed studies may be included, or the analysis may include data from studies that use different methods to measure variables—resulting in a comparison of apples to oranges.

General considerations for judging the validity of a meta-analysis include the following (14):

- *Is the objective clearly stated?*
- *Are the criteria for inclusion or exclusion of studies explicit?*
- *Is the search mechanism for the determination of suitable studies adequate?*
- *Is the quality of the trials included assessed?*
- *Are all of the trials randomized?*
- *Does the discussion include mention of limitations? Does it put results in context?*
- *Are the conclusions justified by the data?*

Summary

This *IFIC Review* presents information to help members of the media, health professionals, and educators critically review food and health-related scientific studies. Such critical review is essential to put the results into the context of the body of scientific literature on a subject and to accurately present the relevance of research to the public.

Although the various elements of a study that have been discussed affect whether a piece of research provides valid and relevant answers to a question being investigated, it is important to realize that "perfect" research does not exist (3). Economics, ethics, and the current state of knowledge may limit a study in its ability to find the answers sought.

Given this, it is also essential to remember that the nature of the scientific process is not linear. It is a process that frequently moves in many different directions, generating questions, discussions, and debates along the way.

How does the communicator maneuver through the maze of emerging scientific findings about food and health to deliver accurate, relevant information to the public? First, by reserving judgment about a study until you have sought out other studies and experts to help assess the findings of the study and their importance—or unimportance. In other words, by putting all research into context. Second, by taking a moderate approach to communicating new information. Realize that what may seem to be a revolutionary, life-altering study today may turn out to be just the opposite tomorrow. That is the nature of research and what makes the journey so exciting.

Key Definitions

Bias—Problems in study design that can lead to effects that are not related to the variables being studied (16). An example is selection bias, which occurs when study subjects are chosen in a way that can misleadingly increase or decrease the strength of an association. Choosing experimental and control group subjects from different populations would result in a selection bias.

Blind, Single or Double—In a single-blind experiment, the subjects do not know whether they are receiving an experimental treatment or a placebo (4). In a double-blind experiment, neither the researchers nor the participants are aware of which subjects receive the treatment until after the study is completed.

Confounding Variable or Confounding Factor—A "hidden" variable that may cause an association that the researcher attributes to other variables (17).

Control Group—The group of subjects in a study to whom a comparison is made to determine whether an observation or treatment has an effect (9). In an experimental study, it is the group that does not receive a treatment. Subjects are as similar as possible to those in the test group.

Correlation—An association, or when one phenomenon is found to be accompanied by another (16). A correlation does not prove cause and effect. Correlation may also be defined statistically.

Experimental Group—The group of subjects in an experimental study that receives a treatment (9). *Generalizability*—The extent to which the results of a study are able to be applied to the general population of people that is comparable to the population studied (18).

Incidence—The number of new cases of a disease during a given period of time in a defined population (6).

Meta-analysis—A quantitative technique in which the results of several individual studies are pooled to yield overall conclusions (6).

Outcomes Research—Type of research that is increasingly used by the health industry and that provides information about how a specific procedure or treatment regimen affects the subject (clinical safety and efficacy), the subject's physical functioning and lifestyle, and economic considerations such as saving or prolonging life and avoiding costly complications (19).

Placebo—Sometimes casually referred to as a "sugar pill," a placebo is a "fake" treatment that seems to be identical to the real treatment (4). Placebo treatments are used to eliminate bias that may arise from the expectation that a treatment should produce an effect.

Prevalence—The number of existing cases of a disease in a defined population at a specified time (6).

Prospective Study—Epidemiological research that follows a group of people over a period of time to observe the potential effects of diet, behavior, and other factors on health or the incidence of disease (4). In general, it is considered a more valid research design than retrospective research.

Randomization, or Random Assignment—A process of assigning subjects to experimental or control groups in which the subjects have an equal chance of being assigned to each group (9). Used to control for known, unknown, and difficult-to-control-for variables.

Random Sampling—A method by which subjects are selected to participate in a study in which all individuals in a population have an equal chance of being chosen (9). Helps to ensure the generalizability of the study results.

Reliability—Whether a test or instrument used to collect data, such as a questionnaire, gives the same results if repeated with the same person several times (20). A reliable test gives reproducible results.

Research Design—How a study is set up to collect information or data (10). For valid results, the design must be appropriate to answer the question or hypothesis being studied. *Residual Confounding*—The effect that remains after one has attempted to statistically control for variables that cannot be measured perfectly (17). This is a particularly important concept in epidemiological studies because knowledge of human biology is still developing. There may exist unknown variables that could significantly change conclusions made on the basis of epidemiological research.

Retrospective Study—Research that relies on recall of past data or on previously recorded information. Often, this type of research is considered to have limitations because the number of variables cannot be controlled and because memory is not infallible (4).

Risk—A term encompassing a variety of measures of the probability of an outcome. It is usually used in reference to unfavorable outcomes such as illness or death (6). Be certain to distinguish between absolute risk and relative risk.

Risk Factor—Anything statistically shown to have a relationship with the incidence of a disease (4). Does not necessarily infer cause and effect.

Statistical Power—A mathematical quantity that indicates the probability a study has of obtaining a statistically significant effect (16). A high power of 80 percent, or 0.8, indicates that the study—if conducted repeatedly—would produce a statistically significant effect 80 percent of the time. On the other hand, a power of only 0.1 means that there would be a 90 percent chance that the research missed the effect—if one exists at all.

Statistical Significance—The probability of obtaining an effect or association in a study sample as or more extreme than the one observed if there was actually no effect in the population (10). On the basis of the hypothesis that if there truly is no effect, the results of a study are unlikely to have occurred. A P value of less than 5 percent (P < 0.05) means that the result would occur less than 5 percent of the time if there were no effect and is generally be considered evidence of a true treatment effect or a true relationship.

Validity—The extent to which a study or study instrument measures what it is intended to measure (20). Refers to accuracy or truthfulness in regard to a study's conclusion.

Variable—Any characteristic that may vary in study subjects, such as gender, age, body weight, diet, behavior, attitude, or other attribute (10). In an experiment, the treatment is called the independent variable; it is the factor being investigated. The variable that is influenced by the treatment is the dependent variable; it may change as a result of the effect of the independent variable.

References

1. Moore M, ed. Health Risks and the Press: Perspectives on Media Coverage of Risk Assessment and Health. Washington, DC: The Media Institute; 1989.

2. Angell M, Kassirer JP. Clinical research—what should the public believe? N Engl J Med. 1994;331(31):189-190.

3. Williams L. Stalking the Elusive Healthy Diet. The New York Times, October 11, 1995.

4. Why do those #&*?@! "experts" keep changing their minds? UC Berkeley Wellness Letter, February 1996.

5. Blonz E. Scientific studies: how to handle the hype. Vegetarian Times, March 1995.

6. Langseth L. Nutritional Epidemiology: Possibilities and Limitations. ILSI Europe Concise Monograph Series; 1996.

7. Charlton BG. Should epidemiologists be pragmatists, biostatisticians, or clinical scientists? Epidemiology 1996;7(5):552-554.

8. Scandlyn JN. How to read a research article. Orthopaed Nurs. 1987;6(5):21-27.

9. Tait PE. Do-it-yourself evaluation of experimental research. J Vis Impair Blindness October 1984;356-363.

10. Schantz D, Lindeman CA. Reading a research article. J Nurs Admin. March 1982;30-33.

11. Dupont W. Converting relative risks to absolute risks: a graphical approach. Stat Med. 1989;8(6):641-651.

12. Savitz D, Olshan A. Multiple comparisons and related issues in the interpretation of epidemiologic data. Am J Epidemiol. 1995;142(9):904-908.

13. Angell M, Kassirer J. Editorials and conflicts of interest. N Engl J Med. 1996;335(14):1055-1056.

14. Geller NL, Proschan M. Meta-analysis of clinical trials: a consumer's guide. J Biopharm Stat. 1996;6(4):377-394.

15. Dattilo A, Kris-Etherton PM. Effects of weight reduction on blood lipids and lipoproteins: a meta-analysis. Am J Clin Nutr. 1992;56(2):320-328.

16. Moore DS. Statistics Concepts and Controversies. New York: W.H. Freeman and Company; 1996.

17. Beecher H. The concept of residual confounding in regression models and some applications. Stat Med. 1992;11:1747-1758.

18. Berkowitz L, Donnerstein E. External validity is more than skin deep: some answers to criticisms of laboratory experiments. Am Psychologist 1982;37(3):245-257.

19. Gallagher-Allred C, Voss A. Nutrition Intervention and Patient Outcomes: A Self-Study Manual. Ross Products Division, Abbott Laboratories, and The American Dietetic Association; 1995.

20. Sherry B. Descriptive epidemiologic research. Monsen ER, ed. In: Research: Successful Approaches. Chicago: The American Dietetic Association; 1992.

7

Your Genetic Signature and Your Food: Debates

Foods Tailored to Your Genotype

According to a University of Auckland, New Zealand press release online at: http://www.crop.cri.nz/home/news/archives/2004/1085626149582.jsp titled, "Research into nutrigenomics opens opportunities for new high-value foods," dated May 27 2004, the science program leader, Professor Lynnette Ferguson from the University of Auckland, is enthusiastic about the potential of diet to make a real difference to genetically-linked diseases.

The article quotes Ferguson as reporting, "We know that a small number of genes may play a disproportionate role in disease development, and that they may be particularly responsive to manipulation by diet. If we can understand the interactions between diet and genes, this will not only help manage disease, but could help us optimize physical and mental performance, slow the effects of aging and reduce health care costs."

The press release also noted that, "An initial focus will be on diseases, such as Crohn's disease, where foods are known to play a role in triggering the genes which cause disease. Later research might focus on the development of foods for use in preventing or managing conditions such as diabetes, obesity and cardiovascular disease, or on optimizing human performance."

Effective screening systems for defective genes also are needed. Other questions also arise. Does a defective gene in one area of the body signal a gene for some benefit in another area of the body? Are functional foods being developed? Will there be an improvement in the quality of life from genetic screening systems? How do genes relate to how people metabolize food or medicine? All these questions are ripe for debate because they relate to issues in nutrition as well as current controversies to be discussed and researched.

What about the issue of individual response to food and medicine leading to personalized medicine and personalized nutrition? Who stands to profit by creating new market opportunities for tailored foods enhanced with specific nutrients? Do different people respond differently to the same food, medicine, or skin-care products? Some people are allergic to some foods. Some people metabolize food differently based on their individual genetic signatures. But, do people respond differently to food, medicines, or anesthesia based on their ethnicities?

Can people with genetic predispositions to diseases take a food-based approach to health? How do we know the way people respond to certain foods when most people have mixed ethnicities over tens of thousands of years? Are there tests that show you how you might respond to a particular food, vitamin, nutrient, medicine, skin-care product, or anesthesia, or what you are allergic to based on your genes? Can response be tested at the molecular level rather than at the racial or ethnic level? Are there smart foods?

Which diseases are notorious for having several genes known to be associated with increased risk? Do studies show that the types of food eaten and the particular environment change the susceptibility of individuals to the disease? All these topics are excellent for debate. Almost everyone is interested in how individuals respond to food.

The goal of nutrigenomics is to develop foods that can be matched to individual human genotypes to benefit the health of those individuals and enhance normal physiological processes. Foods and nutrients influence the genetic control of metabolism. How metabolism is controlled is by through the changing the expression of genes. Exercise, stress and maternal nutrition also have an influence on the individual's response to food or medicine.

Your genotype is defined as genes that any living being (animal, human, or plant) possesses. (Science classifies humans also as animals.) Your phenotype is defined as the observable characteristics of an individual as well as the expression of the genes present in an individual. Your phenotype also is defined as the way your genes are expressed that determines what you are and the way that you perform.

There are many ways that the interplay between your individual genes, what you eat, and the environment can vary. According to a May 27, 2004 University of Auckland, New Zealand press release titled, "*The Science Behind Nutrigenomics,*" animal studies show that the interaction between the environment and genotype can modulate (vary) the expression of individual genes, turning them on or off or regulating the level of expression.

What you might want to debate could be how much do your genes vary? The word 'modulate' stated in the press release also means to vary in tone, inflection, pitch or other quality of sound. For more information, see the entire May 27 2004 press release titled, "*The Science Behind Nutrigenomics,*" which is at: the Crop and Food Research (Auckland University, Auckland, New Zealand), Web site at: http://www.crop.cri.nz/home/news/related-files/1085626149582a.jsp. The sub-title of the press release is: "*Research Into Nutrigenomics Opens Opportunities For New High-Value Foods.*" The purpose of beginning your research with news releases is to guide you to read the abstracts of related medical articles, and then to move on to learning to read the actual medical and scientific articles in journals that you can find in most university libraries.

These libraries usually are open to the public. Some of the most valuable sources for research are the medical school libraries (and university libraries) because of their many scientific journals available to the general public for reading that you may not find at your local public library branch. If you're going to debate, write about, or discuss new findings, visit your local university or medical school library and look at the periodicals.

◆　　　◆　　　◆

How Do Your Genes Respond to Food?

How do your genes respond to what you eat? How many diet-by-DNA book titles are there? Books on smarter foods? Tailored menus? Extracts of plants? DNA tests for ancestry? Ancestry and eating? According to Dr. Fredric D. Abramson, PhD, S.M., President and CEO of *AlphaGenics, Inc.*, Genes are distributed, function, and work in such ways that nearly every reasonable diet could work well in about six percent of the population.

Are you eating smart foods—foods tailored to your genotype—DNA, your ancestry, and your entire genome of genes? Are you ready to get a picture of your response to your nutrition? How can you eat to nourish your genotype? According to Genomics 120, a science, nutrition, and health Web site at: http://g120.com/products/genomicscience.html, are you wondering why in the United States currently only 50,000 people out of some 280 million live to be even 100 years old, or that your body may be aging nearly twice the rate it should be because you're eating the wrong food for your genetic signature?

There is a strong connection between nutrition and genotype, especially in regards to your cardiovascular and central nervous system health. So you need to tailor foods intelligently to your genetic expression. The media buzz about 'intelligent' foods or 'smart' foods really means eating clean, safe, whole foods based on what your individual genes need to thrive. Not all your genes are tested. You might start your food research at the Web site of Food Resource, a source of science-based and business savvy information for the food industry at: http://food.oregonstate.edu/nutri.html.

What happens when diet books for your condition aren't working for you? Maybe salt restriction isn't working but exercise is for your condition. How do your genes respond to nutrition and *nourishment*? Are your genes intelligent, conscious, and communicating with you about their nutritional needs? If they are, so are the foods you eat. Your genes interact and collaborate as a team.

The language of communication is written in the human genome, in your individual genetic signature—in your DNA, in particular SNPs, and in all your genes and cellular material. Even your blood type is expressed in all the cells of your body. How does all this information signal you about what 'smart' foods and nutraceuticals to choose in order to help prevent or delay chronic disease for which your genes may put you at risk?

A slogan reads, "Smart foods for intelligent people." Nutritional genomics is a buzz word in the news. Testing DNA for ancestry also bridges gaps in regard to customizing smarter foods to your genotype. Phenomics is about customized healthcare and medicine tailored to your genetic profile. Prosopography is an independent science of social history embracing genealogy, onomastics and demography. If you're interested in metabolic typing, one Web site for Personal Metabolic Typing is at: http://www.wholebodyhealth.us/. Dentists may be interested to know that gum disease is genetic and may be caused by a genetic predisposition to diabetes, heart disease, or low birth weight. A genetic profile on patients with deep pockets of gum disease might be useful. Check out the Holistic Dental Network at: http://holisticdentalnetwork.com/products_services.php.

Cracking the human genome code is so new and tests so costly. Currently only certain genetic markers are tested. The genetic signatures tested include genes that tell you about risk for certain diseases. Nutritional genomics as a field of research also is abbreviated as a generic term to read 'nutrigenomics.'

Without testing all the genes, how can you know about all the diseases for which you may be at risk? And without knowing all the information that every one of your gene's reveals, how can you develop a plan to override your genetic risks by nourishing your genes with what they need to stay healthier? **Here is how some scientists answered these questions.**

According to Dr. Fredric D. Abramson, PhD, S.M., President and CEO of **AlphaGenics, Inc.**, "The key to using diet to manage genes and health lies in managing gene expression (which we call the Expressitype). Knowing your genotype merely tells you a starting point. Genotype is like knowing where the entrance ramps to an interstate can be found. They are important to know, but tell you absolutely nothing about what direction to travel or how the journey will go. That is why Expressitype must be the focus." You can contact AlphaGenics, Inc. at: http:// www.Alpha-Genics.com or write to: Maryland Technology Incubator, 9700 Great Seneca Highway, Rockville, MD 20850.

Alpha Genics, Inc. is a nutrigenomics science company. A sidebar on the company's Web site from Dr. Fredric Abramson, CEO reads (reprinted here with permission), "We are about to see a revolution in our concept of diet. Each of us is a unique organism and for the first time in human history, genetic research is confirming that one diet is not optimum for everyone.

Science is discovering that each individual's DNA processes food and nutritious supplements in a unique way. Through the development of a cutting-edge DNA analytical system and consumer guidance, Alpha Genics will be able to tune nutrition to meet the needs of each individual resulting in optimum health, peak performance, and enhanced creativity." What I also like about Alpha-Genics Inc. is that they have an independent, separate Ethics Board. Check out that Web site at: http://www.alpha-genics.com/ethics_board.php.

It is not part of the regular Board of Directors. It has five members: three outsiders, one representative from the Board of Directors, and one representative of the employees. The Ethics Board has no veto power, but has a seat on the Board of Directors. Compensation for the Ethics Board members comes through a blind trust, which means the Ethics Board has neither control nor knowledge of how the funds develop.

"I created this because I think companies need to have independent voices to provide reality checks," says Dr. Fredric Abramson. "It is something like that scene in Patton when he talks about the Roman conqueror returning home to glory, with someone standing just beside him reminding him that fame is fleeting. An independent Ethics Board helps us make better choices."

Consumers can bridge the gap between ethics boards and the media by acting as liaisons, ombudsmen, lobbyists, trustees, recruiters, communicators, independent board members, fee-for-service contractors, industry watchers, or volunteers. Get involved in the nutritional genomics industry.

You even can put together corporate gift baskets full of nutritional genomics products or samples. Throw a nutritional genomics party in any home, office, or meeting pace, in church basements, teacher's lounges after school, or at conventions. Make tape recordings about nutritional genomics and post the radio-length broadcasts to your Web site. So many news stories in the media give the impression that the average consumer will have to *wait a decade* for genomic testing to be applied to customized foods.

For example, the New York Times Magazine published an article by NY Times Magazine writer Bruce Grierson titled, "What Your Genes Want You to Eat: New Way to Look at Disease." The article also appeared in the Sacramento Bee, a daily newspaper, on Sunday July 13, 2003 on the Science page. Sundays are great for reading the Science page in the Forum section. There's time to read the cutting-edge science articles, many of which are reprinted from other, major urban publications. It's a family tradition for four decades.

I was impressed by the media buzz around the relatively new field of nutritional genomics. Last year the media buzz circled around testing DNA for ancient ancestry and genealogy, during which I took several DNA tests for ancestry and enjoyed the results. This year DNA and diet is fast-track news. DNA and foods also tie into food safety and security issues.

I like to know that when I go into a health food store and buy a package of imported powdered ginger under the title of herbs or botanicals that it's clean and contains no toxic pesticides, residues, bad bacteria, or unsafe chemicals. I often thought about who inspects these imports and do they rush through, take enough time, or have enough staff? If I buy fresh ginger root, I'm concerned whether it's organic or still full of pesticide residue. On the other hand, who has time to think these thoughts?

It all came rushing back when I went into a health food store last month, walked past an open bin where a child about twelve years old had just put her hand into the couscous, grabbed a fist full of the grain-like pasta, tossed it into her mouth, chewed it, spit it back into her palm and replaced the couscous that she had just spit into her hand, back into the bin with the rest of the grain. Her mother was busy looking at other products.

She didn't realize I was standing beside her ready to take a scoop myself of the oat groats in the next bin. The scoop hit the floor, and she picked it up and replaced it. The cashier was in the front of the store, the manager in the back room. Why couldn't the store change the bins so that nobody else could spit into the grain? When I brought this to the cashier's attention, she shrugged, looked down, and acted as if nothing had happened. I wondered at that instant, if this is how one consumer's word is received, how will the public perceive us?

There's power in numbers, in grouping together. I wished I had my video camera at that moment. There's also power in the media—the reputable, credible media that bridges gaps between science and the public. It's time for some consumers to become "media people." Let's watch the watchers and look at the media.

The article titled, "What Your Genes Want You to Eat: New Way to Look at Disease," had its first opening sentence beginning with a trip to the "'diet doc' circa 2013." I eagerly wanted this kind of testing to be available now, not in 2013. So I turned to Dr. Frederic Abramson, CEO of Alpha-Genics Incorporated to interview by email on his views. Dr. Abramson also teaches part-time at Johns Hopkins University, in the graduate program in Biotechnology.

I asked Dr. Frederic Abramson, CEO of Alpha-Genics Incorporated the following questions in an October 2004 e-interview. Here are his answers.

1. When do you think genomic testing might be available to most consumers?

This is an important question. From a practical perspective, genomic testing—for part of a person's total genome—is possible today. We can test for several thousand genes right now. So this leads to two sub-questions: When will testing of an entire genome become possible? When will low-cost testing be available?

Experts argue about whether we have 30,000 or 70,000 genes, or somewhere in between. Regardless of the number, we are five years away from a comprehensive full genotype test of all genes in a person. By genotype, I mean the identification of which genes a person has.

But it is not your genotype which determines things. It is the work that your specific genes do. Think of genotype as the location of exit ramps on an interstate. You need to know where these are, but they tell you nothing about where you are going and what the journey will be like.

To identify these, we must look at each gene's level of activity, called "gene expression." We call the gene expression the Expressitype. Gene expression changes over time for many genes. How do we know this? Because we age. We start as children, go though puberty, become adults, and then start declining. All of this is substantially under genetic control. Some people age faster than other. It's in their genes.

Right now testing costs a fair amount. And seldom is gene testing covered by insurance. But over time, the technology advances will enable very low cost tests. For example, measuring gene expression in several thousand genes can cost between $800 to $3,000, depending on who does it. But a Japanese company is working on a test that will end up costing less than $100 for 900 genes. Thus, one thing we can be sure of is that the costs will drop. Just like computers, VCR's and microwaves.

We are working to bring the test cost to be under $1,000, with a monthly follow-up of around $79. The monthly fee lets you contact us by phone or email anytime to ask whether something you want to eat might help you or not.

We are working with Carnegie Mellon University in Pittsburgh to develop a small implantable device that will measure vital chemicals in the blood, and send signals outside the body. This will let us track what is happening in a person around the clock, every day, with much more accuracy and less guesswork.

2. What do you think is the most important area of research in nutritional genomics today?

The most important area is to identify how the dietary system, which is composed of hundreds and thousands of chemicals in varying dosages, interacts with the thousands of genes in the genome to produce health, or illness. This is generally called "systems biology." Basically, we can no longer look at single things for easy answers. It won't be just a question of whether you eat blueberries or bananas or rice, but what balance of each of these you eat over time.

This points to the second area, to understand the dynamics of how changes in diet influence the work each person's genes is doing. The value of systems biology is that ultimately, we will be able to identify individualized responses to diet, based on genetic composition.

3. Do you have any advice for those who are looking for tailored diets for specific conditions—if genotype testing is not available today, what is the next best thing for the average consumer who has already had a DNA test of merely the mtDNA or Y chromosome for ancestry?

Ironically, many of the folk suggestions about diet weren't far wrong. So first look to your family history. If you have heart disease in your family, think about a diet that has a bit less fat and more antioxidants. There are similar observations about other conditions like arthritis and cancer.

Generally, if you have a DNA test at this point, it is for one or very few genes. This helps. But remember that most major health conditions are the result of many, many genes acting in concert, not just one gene.

I'll admit it can be confusing with so many different recommendations about diet. To me, this reflects the way in which our genetic diversity makes one diet work well for me and not well for you, while another diet has the exact opposite effect.

4. What is the area of research your company is focusing on now?

Our research focus is to understand how the specific ingredients of diet influence genetic activity. And by diet we include food, supplements, medications, chemicals in water, and even cosmetics, for all of these contain chemicals that influence genes.

The goal of our research is to translate the science into practical day-to-day advice for each person, based on his/her own genetic profile and genetic activity. We want to make genomics something that is useful for each of use every day instead of some industrial science.

This is the same thing that happened when Edison invented the light bulb. Suddenly, electricity was something that every home needed. For us, our success in delivering NutriGenomics to the consumer will make genomics something that everyone will want to use to live their lives a bit better.

5. Where can I refer readers today to learn more?

The amount of literature on the Internet is growing almost daily. Two weeks ago, the commission of the FDA mentioned NutriGenomics in his major speech at Harvard.

We welcome readers to contact us. We are assembling the world's first comprehensive NutriGenomic knowledge base, which we will use to help consumers make better choices. We build our research insights on the actual experience of what real people do.

Our current high priority is a totally new method to prevent viral infections using NutriGenomics. We discovered this in January, and have been working to get government support to conduct this important research. We believe we can develop a way to protect many people from the dangers of certain types of viruses, such as a weaponized flu.

6. Do you work with patients directly or only with their managing physicians or both?

We will work with patients directly and with physicians. When a physician is involved, we will be sure to include the physician in the information loop so the person continues to get the best care.

7. How many genes do you test? Do you prescribe a diet or nutraceuticals based on the results?

In the current stage, we will test about 2,000 genes, mainly for the cardiovascular cluster (cardiovascular disease, diabetes, obesity, hypertension, high cholesterol). The virus testing is planned to be a separate test.

The specific food/supplement recommendations are made directly to the person. These change as the person's genetic activity changes. It would be a mistake to prescribe one type of diet for life. Our genes and bodies don't work that way.

The procedure is simple. We get a sample from you, typically from your cheek lining or blood (if you go to a physician). We identify the genes (genotype) and the amount of genetic activity for each gene (expressitype). We provide you a report summarizing the results. Then, depending on your decision, we will provide you general dietary recommendations based on your genes, or will begin to work with you as often as daily to help you choose what you like to eat.

It is worth noting here that the so-called 'med diet' is based on a month of eating, whereas the USDA model is a daily model. We prefer the monthly approach for the evidence is that eating has a cumulative effect. Another way of saying this is "no one meal will ever hurt you. It is the combination of lots of bad meals that hurts. So knock yourself out."

Fredric D. Abramson, Ph.D., S.M.
President & CEO
AlphaGenics, Inc.
http://www.Alpha-Genics.com

According to Dr. Fredric D. Abramson, Ph.D, S.M., Esq. President and CEO of AlphaGenics, Inc., our genes determine how we respond to our environment. In the industry, nutritional genomics also is abbreviated as 'nutrigenomics.' Let's look at Dr. Abramson's article below titled: *"About NutriGenomics,"* Copyright 2002, 2003. Reprinted here with permission.

About NutriGenomics
Fredric Abramson, Ph.D., S.M., Esq.
Copyright 2002, 2003

Our genes determine who we are, how we develop and age, and how we respond to our environment. They are the blueprints that define our potential. But they do not act in a vacuum. They respond to and actually help shape our environment. That environment includes what we put into our body in food, water, supplements, nutraceuticals and pharmaceuticals.

Together, our genes and environment control our health and our susceptibility to disease. NutriGenomics involves decoding how the molecular composition of our diet, which includes food, supplements, pharmaceuticals and water) influences the work being done by our genes, and then defining personalized dietary strategies to tune each person's gene expression pattern, called the "Expressitype." This tuning process must be changed dynamically as the person's genetic activity changes.

"NutriGenomics lets people pick the foods they eat based on how well the foods make their genes function."

Because what we eat influences our health and the way our genes work, we have the opportunity to let people control their health destiny in a whole new way. This is what NutriGenomics is about: calibrating the mix and amounts of what ingredients we put into our body so that our genes work at their best, for our best health status. By building on each person's genetic uniqueness, NutriGenomics focuses on what that individual's genes are doing and how that person can pick and choose things from their environment that will make his/her genes work better or worse.

AlphaGenics approach is to identify what parts of your diet are making your genes work badly, and determine the best mixture in your diet to calibrate and tune the work your genes are doing. Our goal is to adjust your genetic activity, without changing your genes, by dynamically adjusting the mix of what you put into your body as your body changes over time.

Basic Terms

▶ **Genotype**: The entire set of genes of an individual.
▶ **Expressitype**: The profile of gene expression activity in an individual at a moment in time.
▶ **Phenotype**: The observable characteristics of an individual.
▶ **NutriGenomics**: The science that relates how the molecular inputs from a person's environment influence and control gene expression.
▶ **Qwink**: A molecule or particle in the environment that can change gene expression directly or indirectly.
▶ **Expressitype Knowledge Transfer System**: A proprietary information/knowledge management system that integrates individual longitudinal data with a variety of scientifically verified data elements. Its outputs include personalized, dynamic dietary strategies as well as a variety of scientific and research-oriented solutions.

Our dietary environment influences how our genes work

Many different ingredients exist in a person's dietary environment. They exist as both natural molecules and artificial compounds and are found in food as well as in our water, and in dietary supplements, cosmetics and medications. Even in the air we breathe. Some are present by design; others as a by-product. So, for example, the common tomato is known to have over 300 different natural molecules. Some ingredients are man-made, but most are natural substances whose variety and health-effects are not even fully explored.

The key to NutriGenomics is identifying how specific compounds or chemicals in our diet influence the activity of one or more genes, and hence our health.

Our focus is on our genetic activity (Expressitype) and not just what genes we have (Genotype). Knowing your genotype is a lot like knowing where the entrance is to an interstate highway. It is very useful and important, but it doesn't tell you what direction to go in or when you will be able to stop for gas.

The term "Qwink" was coined to refer to any molecule in the dietary stream that influences gene expression. Qwinks are found in foods, supplements, cosmetics, water and pharmaceutical compounds. They include basic ingredients such as sugars, proteins and fat as well as very specialized substances such as vitamins or toxins. A Qwink may be a natural substance or synthetic.

A Qwink is neutral as to whether it has a positive or negative effect. If the gene expression moves in the direction to provide better health or reduce risk, it is good; if it moves to worsen a person's health status, it is bad. Thus, it is only the effects that are good or bad. For example, a pesticide residue that survives in the food chain and influences gene expression is a Qwink.

While pesticides are generally considered harmful, interestingly enough, there is some evidence that certain pesticides could actually reduce the risk of cancer, at least in model systems.[1]

NutriGenomics calibrates dietary inputs and patterns to provide different Qwink types and concentrations to the genetic machinery.

The impact of a Qwink typically depends on its concentration and dosage frequency.

One of the amazing aspects of human biology is that it responds differently to varied Qwink concentrations. Take arsenic, for example. Most people know that arsenic in high doses can kill. What is less commonly known, however, is that at very low concentrations, arsenic is considered a nutrient.

The same will be found for how Qwinks work. At very low concentrations, one set of genes may be affected while a much higher concentration may change expression in an entirely different set of genes.

NutriGenomics is personalized genomics

The way a person's dietary environment influences gene expression and health is called NutriGenomics. NutriGenomics is a scientific platform that permits focused personalized adjustments to a person's dietary environment. An advantage of NutriGenomics is that it is a unifying standard that includes the effect of dietary supplements, nutraceuticals, pharmaceuticals and cosmetics in addition to what a person normally eats, as well as environmental factors such as toxins, contaminants and infectious agents, such as viruses and bacteria. The scientific goal is to identify molecular levers coming from a person's environment that can move the person's gene expression patterns in an appropriate direction, and to further identify environmental adjustments that can help improve the person's health status through changes in gene expression.

Our core scientific proposition is that evaluating and modulating a person's Expressitype as it dynamically changes over time is a more potent and acceptable way to prevent and control disease than working with genotype alone. The practical difference between focusing on genotype versus expressitype is comparable to the difference between buying a car based on what Consumer Reports says is

---

1.   John Milner, National Cancer Institute, personal communication, January 2003.

its repair frequency and listening to your car coughing and sputtering when you are driving down the highway.

The cycle begins with a person's environment, which interacts with the person's genotype and can up-regulate or down-regulate various genes. The gene expression pattern, the expressitype, in turn, works to produce proteins and otherwise control the person's metabolism and physiology to produce the phenotype. It is a person's phenotype at which we observe health and illness. Examples of phenotype include eye color, blood groups, and various chronic and acute diseases. A person's phenotype in turn helps shape the environment. For example, phenotype can influence what a person chooses to eat. A person who doesn't feel well may eat differently; a person who changes their physical activity may also change how they eat; and so on.

AlphaGenics designed its research and intervention around this cycle. By capturing data and information from each individual, including serial measures of expressitype, and blending this data with scientific knowledge from genomics, nutrition, pharmacology, toxicology, and medicine, we can focus on unraveling the systems biology map of how the complex environment interacts with and influences the comparably complex genome.

Our genome works as a system that takes us through our life cycle

Our genetic apparatus is a complex system designed to sustain our lives in intimate communication with the environment, from birth through puberty and the gradual aging process leading to the end of our lives. It is this complexity that has made it so difficult to find cures or treatments for so many diseases like cancer and heart disease. It is this same complexity that explains why a drug will work in one person, be ineffective in another, and harm a third. It is this complexity that confirms why different people need entirely different diets to lose weight, for example.

The fact is also that almost all of the major health conditions that concerns society today—cancer, heart disease, diabetes, obesity, neurological and similar disorders are all multifactorial and polygenic. Multifactorial means that it is both environment and genetics in combination that explains when, why and where different diseases occur. Polygenic means that multiple genes are involved, not just one.

Three specific aspects of this complexity are worth exploring. First, the number of different genes involved with each of the diseases that plague us can be in the hundreds or even thousands. Second, virtually every chemical that we put into our body influences some genes. And third, our genes typically work collaboratively, where one influences another. Our genes work as an integrated, cohesive system.

A change in gene expression is not always a benefit

The goal of NutriGenomics is to move gene expression patterns to some "best" state. However, because the human genome is complex, an important issue is that an "increase or a decrease" in gene expression is not "always" linked with a benefit. A lot may depend on what the other genes involved are doing as well.

Many different genes are involved in the common health conditions

Most of the common conditions that concern our health are polygenic, i.e. involve many different genes as mentioned above. The goal of the Human Genome Project was to identify thousands of genes and to link these genes to specific health effects. Scientists are also pinpointing exactly where each of these genes are located, or "mapped," on our chromosomes.[2]

Some examples include breast cancer (over 200 genes, 39 of which are mapped to 17 different chromosomes), obesity (over 200 genes; 15 mapped to 11 chromosomes); Diabetes (60 mapped genes to 17 different chromosomes); Lymphoma (200 mapped genes on 22 chromosomes); and hypertension (19 genes on 10 chromosomes).[3]

Qwinks impact multiple genes, not just one

What we put into our body typically influences more than one gene. For example, the natural compound retinoic acid can change expression in more than 500 different genes[4] while the enzyme Cofactor Q10 will up- or down-regulate over 100 different genes.[5]

Genes work together as a coherent system, not as independent actions.

For a polygenic condition, it is important to realize that the genes involved do not work by themselves but work in a coherent, structured system. We can take as an example the more than 200 different genes implicated in obesity. If each of

---

2.   Humans have 22 pairs of chromosomes plus the X and Y.
3.   Obtained from the Human Genome Project web site.
4.   Balmer and Blomhoff, Gene Expression Regulation by Retinoic Acid, Journal of Lipid Research, Vol. 43, 1773-1808 (November 2002).
5.   Linnane AW, et al. Cellular redox activity of CoQ10:effect of Q10 supple. On human skel. muscle. Free Rad Res 2002;36(4):445-453.

these genes worked independently of one another, there would be 2 to the 200th power different combinations. This is 1.6 times ten to the 60th power; that is, 1.6 followed by 60 zeros. This number, 1.6 times ten to the 60th, is very large. In fact, it is larger than all the humans who have ever lived on the earth. It is larger than all the organisms, including viruses that have ever lived on the earth.

So clearly, just by observing that different groups or types exist in obesity, one realizes that these 200 genes don't work independently. In fact, what must happen is that when one gene turns on, it in turn regulates ten or twenty others. This interaction among our genes leads to a relatively small, countable number of combinations of gene activity. Instead of the astronomic number calculated above, we have only 100's or 1000's of combinations for this example of obesity. These combinations are the "typical" patterns of gene activation, so to speak the molecular bar codes, each of which could be associated with a form of the disease.

So it is possible to imagine two type of obese people, one with five obesity genes turned on, say numbers 1, 50, 95, 150 and 200, and the rest turned off; the second with twelve different obesity genes turned on. These two different combinations could translate into different obesity effects, where one type of person gains weight easier than the other on the same diet.

While our genes are fixed at birth, the work they do changes as we age

Each person is born with genes they inherited from their parents. The identity of your genes is called the "Genotype." The Genotype is a person's unique collection of genes. Classic genetics described genotypes for hair and eye color, and blood types. For all practical purposes, the genotype is fixed when your parents' sperm and egg unite.

Genes are dynamic engines. Their work varies depending on circumstances and time. The entire genomic system changes its work, as illustrated by the aging process that begins with infancy, moves through childhood, puberty and adulthood, and then to senescence. These genetic mechanisms are starting to be understood.

An example of gradual, almost invisible changes in genetic activity is observed in how menstrual cycles shorten as a woman ages. Research done at the University of Minnesota in the 40's shows that a 40 year old woman has one more menstrual period a year than a 20 year old, and that the one-day per year change in cycle length is linear from 20 to 40. This gradual change suggests that key genetic components to target in NutriGenomics are genes whose activity undergoes very gradual changes over a long time period. This further suggests that many key NutriGenomic interventions will be based on cumulative effects.

It's Gene Expression (Expressitype) Which is Key

The accomplishments of the Human Genome Project mean we will soon be able to identify every gene in a person, in effect, that person's genetic blueprint. Some of these genes will indicate greater risks for certain diseases; other genes will mean less risk than average. An example is the BRCA1 gene for breast cancer. Women with BRCA1 have a significantly higher risk of developing breast cancer than those without it.

The genotype, however, is only a starting place to understand what our genetic destiny might be. This is because the work a gene does is likely to change over time, both according to preprogrammed rules, and in response to environmental influences, notably our food. Some genes are turned on early in life, say during pregnancy, and are switched off permanently. Other genes may just sit there waiting to be activated or to become phenotypically manifest. This appears to be the case with certain diseases that arise later in life, such as Huntington's chorea, a single dominant gene disorder that shows itself in a person's 50's.

Further complicating the situation is that when a gene is "on" it may be operating at one activity level one day and a higher or lower level the next day. A gene's activity is exhibited as "genetic expression," a term that refers to the gene producing RNA and otherwise interacting with a person's metabolism and physiology.

Let's call, in analogy to Genotype, the entire profile of expression of each gene throughout the genome, the "Expressitype." Thus, for any health condition, each person has his or her own Expressitype. The Expressitype is the actual amount of genetic activity produced by each gene that is implicated in or related to a specific health status or condition.

Since for any particular gene that is turned on, the expression level may be changing over time, and because the gene itself may be turned on or off at a particular point in time, a person's Expressitypes is likely to change.

A person's NutriGenomic profile, then, measures what each gene is doing at a point in time. By stringing together a series of NutriGenomic profiles, it is possible to see whether a gene is changing, the direction a gene is going and how fast it is getting there.

The gene-environment interaction is very powerful

The interaction between genes and environment is undisputed. Part of the environment is dietary—what we eat. Another part is lifestyle—how we live our everyday lives. Figure 1 is a general overview of NutriGenomics, starting with the dietary inputs at the base and moving through the genome to the end result of health or illness.

Even well defined genetic disorders respond to environment differences. For example, if identical twins each have the single dominant gene for Huntington's chorea, and the twins have different dietary and exercise programs, the onset of Huntington's chorea can be delayed up to eight years in one of the twins.

Diet has been shown to alter gene expression in several ways Qwinks can act on how DNA is transcribed into RNA They can be involved in various metabolic pathways and can increase or decrease the concentrations of other materials needed by the genome. In other words, Qwink effects can be direct, by changing gene activity itself, or indirect by shifting what is available for the gene to use.

Foods, supplements and other chemical sources are the foundation of NutriGenomics. The ingredients that actively regulate the genome, the Qwinks, can turn genes on and off, and can change the amount of activity for each turned-on gene. The Qwinks help determine the Expressitype, which is the profile of what each gene is doing at a moment in time. Gene expression becomes translated into health, wellness or illness through a person's metabolism and the many proteins in the proteome. Moreover, a person's health status, in turn, influences gene activity and can even change what might be acceptable to eat. An example would be creating an immune response to a certain food (i.e., strawberries) that makes the food dangerous. This system is dynamic, and changes over time as we age and our health changes. Tying these all together are the many biochemical, physiological and metabolic processes with cells and tissues.

◆   ◆   ◆

Genovations™

Let's profile another company that helps you eat better by revealing disease risks, so your physician can concentrate on focused prevention and treatment tailored to your individual genetic signature. Today, there are companies such as *Genovations*™.

According to Marketing Communications at the North-Carolina-based Great Smokies Diagnostic Laboratory, the company approaches preventive health care by using genetic analysis to provide individuals and their physicians with critical information to more effectively control present and future health. Genovations uses information stored in each person's genes to reveal disease risks and to help each individual lead a healthier life though focused prevention and individualized treatment.

Genes provide the key to a wealth of information unique to each individual that, once unlocked, can serve as a comprehensive guide to a healthier life. By identifying specific genetic risk factors and changes in dietary, lifestyle, nutritional supplements and medications that are most likely to improve each patient's health, Genovations enables physicians to practice truly individualized preventive medicine.

Most consumers will ask about what happens when you go for a genetic test. It's more than the DNA test you might have taken to look at your mtDNA or Y-chromosome for deep ancestry. Instead, the kind of genetic testing you'd take at Genovation, for example is to evaluate specific portions of your genetic code.

Genovations™ testing evaluates specific portions of the genetic code that vary from person to person. These variations are called single nucleotide polymorphisms, or SNPs (pronounced "snips") for short. Everyone has SNPs—they're what make people different from one another—our hair color, our height, our voice, even key aspects of our personality. SNPs are the very seat of our individuality. SNPs also affect our health.

Some SNPs can make people more susceptible or more resistant to common diseases. Others may make the body respond differently to certain diets or lifestyle habits.

Read the *Complete Blood Type Diet Encyclopedia*. What nutritional genomics needs is a complete human genome diet dictionary. With 40,000 or more genes in each person shuffling with each generation, individuals inherit different genotypes. At the same time, some abnormal genes are inherited and make members of some families more at risk than other families.

◆   ◆   ◆

Here is an e-letter from Kay Patrick, Product Manager, Genovations.

From: Kay_Patrick
To: 'Anne Hart'
Sent: Tuesday, July 22, 2003 6:46 AM
Subject: RE: Thanks. Just a few questions

Dear Anne:

I have attempted to answer your questions. Please let me know if you have additional questions.

Why are Genovations tests only available through a physician?

Genomic test results are most meaningful and best understood when they are clinically interpreted within the context of a patient's complete health history. For this reason, genomic testing is best managed by a licensed health care professional.

Genovations tests are available only through trained, licensed health care practitioners. Not all practitioners are adequately trained to interpret and use the genomic information revealed in these tests, so Genovations has taken a leading role in providing genomic medical education to health care practitioners.

What does Genovations™ testing do?

Genovations testing focuses only on SNPs in the genetic code that are associated with common health conditions, such as heart disease, osteoporosis, allergies and asthma, for which simple treatment strategies exist to reduce risk. Testing also evaluates SNPs that affect how each person's body is likely to respond to specific diets, supplements, and medications.

Therapeutic recommendations based upon the genetic results are provided for the practitioner to develop a treatment protocol. In this way, test results can provide the physician with a "road map" for developing a comprehensive, personalized health action plan for each patient.

Example:

Heart Disease
MYTH: All persons with a family history of heart disease can minimize their cardiovascular risk by reducing their dietary intake of fat and salt, exercising more, and taking a cholesterol lowering medication.

REALITY: Heart disease is not simply a condition caused by excess fat and cholesterol. Research has revealed that there are many other modifiable risk factors, some genetically influenced that can predispose a person to heart disease.

For example, some people have a genetic inability to properly metabolize folic acid in the body. This can lead to a build-up of homocysteine in the bloodstream, causing increased risk of blood clots and atherosclerosis. Yet none of the "one-size-fits-all" conventional therapies listed above would reduce this risk. For a person with this genetic variation, the only way to reduce risk is to take the active form of folic acid, which is not found in common vitamin supplements.

High blood pressure is typically treated by restricting an individual's salt intake. However, not all people have the genetic variation (a single nucleotide polymorphism, or SNP-pronounced "snip") that allows them to respond effectively to a salt-restricted diet. Based on their genetic make-up, they may respond better to aerobic exercise. By testing genetic variations, the physician can better identify which therapy is likely to be the most effective for lowering blood pressure in each patient.

Apo E is a protein in the body that affects cholesterol levels. There are three major genetic variations of the Apo E gene that can affect how each person's body breaks down fat and cholesterol in the diet. These three variations can lead to an increased, average, or decreased risk of heart disease. By knowing an individual's Apo E genetic variation, the physician can prescribe the dietary and lifestyle changes, nutritional supplements, or prescription medications most likely to lower cholesterol levels effectively.

What is the process?

Practitioners incorporate genomic testing into their complete work-up along with other phenotypic diagnostic tests. Blood samples are collected in the office, shipped to our laboratory, tested here in our genomics lab and the reported results are shipped back to the ordering practitioner who schedules a follow-up with the patient.

How much does a Genovations test cost?

The cost of Genovations testing depends on the testing option chosen by the patient and the practitioner. The comprehensive testing program, which assesses health risks for a wide range of conditions (including heart disease, osteoporosis, and immune dysfunction) costs about $1,000-$2,000. Focused testing for health risks associated with a single area or condition costs about $300-$500.

Hope that helps.

Sincerely,
Kay Patrick

Product Manager, Genovations
www.genovations.com

◆   ◆   ◆

An overview of what genes are, how they are inherited, and how many are in the human body is presented on the Web site at: http://www.genovations.com/patient_overview.html. What can testing a small number of genes actually reveal about how your body processes specific foods and medicines?

What Can SNPs Tell You About Your Genotype?

SNPs can even affect whether certain drugs are likely to have severe side effects or not. By evaluating these health-related SNPs, Genovations™ testing allows physicians to develop preventive strategies that are tailored to each patient's unique genetic makeup and health risks. This helps to reduce the guesswork that results from using "one-size-fits-all" approach to preventive medicine.

Genovations™ is a line of tests that is only available for a licensed health care provider (doctor) to order for a patient. The test results are provided directly to the health care provider, who consults with his or her patient.

Genovations does not interpret test results for the patient or the health care provider. A patient's health care provider uses the test result information to determine appropriate treatment protocols for the patient. Genovations™ does not provide specific nutriceuticals or supplements recommendations. That is up to the health care provider.

According to marketing communications, "Genovations does not test for SNPs. We currently have 4 profiles that identify specific SNPs related to heart disease, detoxification problems, bone health, and immunology related problems. Each profile identifies between 7 and 15 SNPs."

If you want more information about Genovations, write to them, email them, or telephone. Genovations' phone number and email address are listed at its Web site. Since books hang around libraries for years, but phone numbers may or may not change, you can reach Great Smokies Diagnostic Laboratory or Genovations™ as follows: Corporate Headquarters, Great Smokies Diagnostic Laboratory/Genovations™ 63 Zillicoa Street, Asheville, NC 28801, USA

Or go to their Web sites at: http://www.genovations.com/ and/or at: www.gsdl.com. See the Web site at: http://www.gsdl. com/assessments/finddisease/cardiovascular/metabolic glycemia.html.

Read about metabolic glycemia. If you have insulin resistance, or too much insulin pouring out every time you eat certain carbohydrates, you'd want to read more about this and how it changes or affects your arteries and other parts inside your body.

There are excellent sites on the Web to educate yourself before you decide to get tested. Check out your biomarkers. Before you see your doctor, know what questions to ask and what tests to ask for. Then talk it over with your physician.

When you take control over what you eat you are educating yourself as to your body's nutritional requirements to maintain health, stay fit, and prevent or delay chronic illness at any age. Your genetic profile tells you how your genes are responding to the food you eat.

With 30,000, 40,000, or 70,000 genes in each individual and each person inheriting a different genotype, you'd need a customized diet book for each person on Earth. Each individual's genetic signature is different.

Nobody responds exactly the same way to certain foods. That's why genetic testing helps to *customize* food plans for the individual. Some people have allergies. Others respond to foods gradually and silently inside their arteries and organs.

Intelligent Foods

Another buzz word in the media is 'smart' or 'intelligent' foods—foods tailored to your genetic signature. It's not that the food is smart or genetically changed. It's that the food in a relatively unprocessed, natural, clean state is free from vermin, full of life and enzymes. That prescribed food according to the person's gene expression is then healthier to eat for that particular person. Another person could be allergic to it and become sicker.

The food itself is freer of toxins. Additionally, the 'smart' or 'intelligent' food terminology really means the *act of tailoring or customizing the food to the person's genetic profile*. It does not mean the food is genetically altered and may or may not be dangerous to humans. 'Intelligent' foods refer to the results of your genetic testing.

You're the person being smarter by eating what the results of genetic tests reveal. The results are interpreted by a professional. In addition, you need to find out for yourself how to apply the test results to what happens to you when you eat a particular food combination or take a certain group of nutraceuticals.

In making a food such as raw soy milk, for example, you need to know that raw soy can take certain nutrients out of your body if the soy milk is not cooked for a certain length of time before it is bottled, cooled and then consumed. Blue, purple, and red-colored fruit or vegetables are excellent for your health, if your genotype says so. Eating raw blue berries also will take out certain vitamins from your body unless the berries are frozen or cooked.

You need to know how to process raw vegetables and fruits either by cooking and/or freezing before they are consumed so that eating them day after day in certain amounts won't lead to the leaching out of various vitamins, enzymes, or minerals from your body. Knowledge is important here. When you are prescribed certain foods, make sure you know how to prepare them for the maximum nutrient benefits.

Diets need to be tailored to individuals. There are only four blood types, but individual genotypes are different for each person. You'd need a customized diet book for each person on Earth. Each individual's genetic signature is different. Nobody responds exactly the same way to certain foods. That's why genetic testing helps to customize food plans for the individual. Some people have allergies. Others respond to foods gradually and silently inside their arteries and organs.

Not only do people of different ethnicities react differently to the same doses of medicines, but people of different ethnicities react differently to certain foods. It's touchy to bring in the term "race," but studies have found that people of a certain race react differently to certain drugs for certain conditions, and that people of another race react differently to the same dosage given to another race.

You can read in medical journal articles for example, on how African Americans respond to glaucoma drugs compared to Caucasian people. Read about how the same dose of a drug given to an East Asian and a non-East Asian will be too high a dose for the East Asian.

What about foods? Do people from Northern Europe tolerate milk better than people from Southern Europe? Do many people from Southeast Asia hardly tolerate milk? There is always the exception. People are of mixed ancestry. What you need to learn about is *the ways in which intelligent foods work with your genes.*

You don't know who will react in which ways at the genetic level to the food or medicine or whether the dosage of the drug or the amount of the food will be tolerated or too high or low. Even with varying dosages of nutraceuticals—supplements such as vitamins, food extracts, and minerals, some people benefit and others show no change. Read the results of conflicting studies in medical articles.

If the dosage of vitamins is hotly debated, drug dosages and ethnicity is another topic in the research arena.

Some people have inherited risks for certain chronic diseases. Those people need to eat foods and perhaps take nutritional supplements that will prevent or delay the onset of those problems. Nutritional genomics fills an important need in maintaining health and quality of life. From the ***Institute of Food Research (IFR)*** in Norwich, UK, **Dr. Ruan Elliot, lead IFR scientist,** sent me this e-letter in response to my questions about what is being researched there. Here's the reply.

Dear Anne:

My main research interests are in using so-called functional genomic techniques to define mechanisms by which diet and specific components of the diet promote human health. These powerful techniques are set to revolutionise the way we approach fundamental nutrition research. On top of this, as you will appreciate, there is also the aspect of inter-individual genetic variation, the impact that this has on health and the potential variations in optimal dietary requirements.

To my mind, these two areas are locked together. We need to properly understand the processes by which components of the diet (nutrients, and micronutrients) work individually and together to keep us healthy so as to be able properly to define optimal nutrition for sub-populations or individuals properly based on their genetics.

You can find descriptions of my work and research interests at the following URLs;
http://www.ifr.ac.uk/public/FoodInfoSheets/EDPgenomics.html,
http://bmj.com/cgi/reprint/324/7351/1438.pdf

I hope this is helpful.

Best regards,

Ruan Elliott

For further information, contact the Institute of Food Research, Norwich Research Park, Colney, Norwich NR4 7UA, UK. To view their Web site, phone and fax numbers or email address, on the Internet, go to: http://www.ifr.ac.uk/about/.

My philosophy about genetic testing is to remember a quote by Richard Feynman, Nobel Laureate: "The best way to predict the future is to invent it." Your genes are hard-wired for certain foods, but not all foods make compatible software. Consumers need a guide book to nutritional genomics. You'll hear terms such as gene expression, genetic signatures, risk, intelligent foods, and tailoring the food to your genotype. What it all means is that your body is looking for customized nourishment.

If you really want to take charge of your own health and nutrition, learn all that you can possibly find out about how to apply the results of your DNA testing, genotype testing, metabolic, blood, ancestry, racial percentages testing, and body chemistry or allergy testing to what you eat, the nutraceuticals and supplements you select, your exercise style and lifestyle. Everything starts at the cellular level, even the way your body reacts to stress and exercise with cortisol or with relaxation. Individuals react to certain types of exercise, foods, or perceived stress situations differently.

Some nutrients, foods, herbal compounds or other supplements cause relaxation in some people and panic attacks in others. Then there are allergies to consider. It starts with an expression of your genes in reaction to the environment. Some people get an increase in ocular pressure from sleeping on pillows containing a stuffing to which they are allergic.

One sip of caffeine can start a panic reaction in one person and relaxation in another. Your reaction is in your genes. It's about body type, another genetic expression, whether you have inherited genes for anxiety of certain lengths, and the whole interplay and interface of one team of genes with another group in your body. I refer to this interplay of genes as a "rhumba of rattlesnakes" at the molecular level.

You have a part to play in all this, and it isn't always as the passive patient or recipient. You have the *genomer* and the *genomee*.... Be the *genomer* for a change—the person in the driver's seat. Take control. Take charge of how to interpret your DNA tests for risk and diet changes or for ancestry and family history or for any other purpose for which you want to test your genome or any region of your genetic profile. To be able to understand how to read and interpret a DNA test and apply it to foods and supplements and to know how the foods will actually effect your genetic expression—that kind of knowledge is power.

The information is publicly available in medical school libraries, on the Internet's scientific databases, and in various journals in the nutrition and genetics fields. Most of these sources are open to the public without you having to be a scientist to learn about how your body responds to food at the cellular level.

Start by joining various online groups, visiting your library, and reading the latest medical and scientific journal articles in the field of nutritional genomics. Contact and network with patient support groups using genetic testing. Start your own email list message board for consumers who want to learn and listen in addition to sharing resources of information.

The consumer's role is to compare, review, and find out who is best qualified to work with an individual's genes. How does a consumer discern between snake-oil and reputable companies in this growing field? Who is qualified? Consumers need an explanation in plain language what is healthy to eat, not for the world, but for the individual. So it's up to the consumer to do some research and learn a lot more about nutritional genomics.

Beyond food what does an individual's gene expression require in terms of exercise and lifestyle? It's time to educate your body about nutritional genomics and about DNA and ancestry. What foods should you eat and what nutritional supplements (nutraceuticals) would benefit your health? One way to tell is to test your genetic markers. Which genetic markers? The entire genome? Or specific SNPs that signal risk of certain chronic diseases? Nutritional genomics should be available to all consumers, not only those with money to pay for expensive testing. Sure, in the future the price of genetic testing will come down, but senior citizens and parents today want to know what they can eat that will agree with them and their families.

Researching the Web under "nutritional genomics" I found a company in the United Kingdom called Sciona. According to Sciona's Web site at: http://www.sciona.com/coresite/index.asp?p=1, Sciona is a venture capital backed company that researches and develops tests for common variations in genes which affect your individual response to medicines, food and the environment.

There are around 40,000 genes in the human genome. Sciona identifies those genes that influence a certain function such as cardiovascular status and tests for these as a set or 'panel'. This information is then used by appropriately qualified practitioners to provide you with health advice.

Testing of specific genes rather than the entire genome usually is done by various companies at this time. In the future, the number of genes tested may increase, or science may find which particular genes interact with other genes to put you at risk if you eat certain foods, or whether your specific genes work together in such a way that you can eat almost anything without developing chronic diseases.

According to Sciona's Web site testing specific genes for certain chronic illnesses is useful in guiding aspects of the treatment of diseases such as heart disease and osteoporosis, which are influenced by your genes, lifestyle and environment. For the consumer, knowing which foods to eat to influence your gene expression is important.

According to Sciona's Web site, Sciona's team of geneticists, molecular biologists, medical doctors and dieticians work with universities and other companies to identify the significant genes underlying a particular effect. The effects of these, and other factors such as your diet, are then analyzed to give you specific advice on courses of action tailored to your own genetic makeup and circumstances.

Filling out questionnaires allow consumers to think in terms of focus sheets. Besides DNA testing, food choices, and consultations with your physician, you need to focus on your habits and think how realistically you answer a questionnaire. Think about from which direction you want to participate in nutritional genomics—marketing, research, science, consumer awareness, forming support groups, media, or other. What are your basic interests and how can you apply them to this field? You can contact Market America, Inc. at 1302 Pleasant Ridge Road, Greensboro, NC 27409. Their Web site is at: http://www. marketamerica.com.

Here is an e-letter from Andy Aldridge, Public Relations Director, Market America, Inc.

Dear Anne:

After extensive market surveying and testing, Market America and Cellf, a division of Sciona, have partnered together to offer the Nutri-Physical™ Gene SNP DNA Screening Analysis program. This product allows consumers to submit a sample of their DNA to have it analyzed.

Once the analysis is complete, consumers receive a report that outlines possible deficiencies along with lifestyle and diet changes that can be carried out to address possible vulnerabilities. To accompany the DNA analysis, Market America also developed a questionnaire that, when analyzed in conjunction with the Gene SNP product, results in a suggested list of customized vitamins and supplements, available in one formula, if desired by the consumer.

The company's Isotonix® Custom Formula makes choosing the correct nutritional supplementation a simple and efficient process. From a Distributor Custom Web Portal, a customer submits answers to a dietary and lifestyle questionnaire and has the option of purchasing a unique custom formula nutraceutical that specifically addresses their individual needs.

Many companies are talking about NutriGenomics. Through our partnership with Cellf for DNA analysis and Garden State Nutritionals for manufacturing and customization, we are actually doing it.

Regards,

Andy Aldridge
Public Relations Director
Market America, Inc.

8

Quality Control

You need a voice in quality control. What the consumer needs to understand are the roles of genes in healthcare, and how the *roles of genes* interact when you take in nutrition. Consumers, corporations, venture capitalists the government, taxpayers, and research institutions invest billions of dollars each year to develop this understanding. One example of a consumer group involved in quality control is when parents group together to form their own DNA bank, recruit people to donate DNA for research, and develop databases and Web sites disseminating information on a particular genetic condition.

Consumers can don few or many hats in nutritional genomics. There are avenues to explore varying from watchdog, marketing, research, public relations, parenting, safety, event planning, publishing, gerontology, videography, genealogy, healthcare, to broadcasting.

If you do your research, you'll find that venture capitalists who in the last decade invested heavily in the computer industry are now looking to invest in biotechnology. The power of gene technology drums up business and communication also for patent attorneys, journalists, and inventors.

To participate in nutritional genomics in a variety of capacities as a consumer, you can write to the United States Food & Drug Administration (FDA), Department of Agriculture (USDA), and National Institutes of Health (NIH), as well as university laboratories, pharmaceutical manufacturers, and government agencies worldwide. Get involved in the power of genetic technology at some level. The FDA is the agency that's responsible for 80 percent of the United States food supply, according to a July 1st 2003 speech given by the Commissioner, Food and Drug Administration.

In that July 1, 2003 speech before Harvard School of Public Health, Mark B. McClellan, MD, PhD, Commissioner, Food and Drug Administration, said, "All of you—consumer advocates, representatives of the food industry, nutrition scientists, and other food experts—have a collective commitment to the issues we face at FDA that is integral to our ability us fulfill our mission. And your help is needed more than ever. Now more than ever, we all must work together to find better solutions."

It's important to read this speech and to look at materials on the Web at the Harvard School of Public Health. Click on the Harvard School of Public Health's Web site at: http://www.hsph.harvard.edu/now/jul11/conference.html. Read the important facts there and check out the forums. The current headline at the Web site notes that "A July 2003 conference at the Harvard School of Public Health 'spurred' dialogue with the nation's food industry on the subject of "'Changing the American Diet' To Improve Health." Read the materials there and think for yourself about how the food you eat is processed and marketed.

In the speech, you'll find key words such as "consumer advocates" and "collective commitment." Your help indeed is needed to work together as a team, to share, with a purpose of finding better solutions. That's why it's important to listen and learn all you can about the future of nutritional genomics. The consumer's involvement is important. The theme emphasized "collaborating to improve the American diet." Collaborating with consumers also means working to decrease obesity and epidemics of diabetes in children.

You can look at the American diet from the point of view of those who work in DNA testing, from those who work with family history and ancestry research, or from those who work in food packaging and processing. It really hits home when you look from the point of view of the consumer or from marketing and product management. Everybody has to eat.

Surveillance

There's another branch of nutritional genomics that instead of only testing your DNA to find out which foods are healthiest for your genes, focuses on *manipulating plant micronutrients* to improve human health. See the article on the Internet, a PDF file on a Web site at: **http://www.ipef.br/melhoramento/genoma/pdfs/ dellapenna99.pdf.**

The volume of imported food is growing each year. Consumers have a field cut out for them—surveillance. As FDA increases its examinations and sampling at borders, consumers can work together to research information about food imports and inspection.

A laboratory can only sample so many products. Consumers can take a role in food security, perhaps looking at industry to identify problems or threats. What the consumer's role entails is better information and collaboration. Everyone needs to keep costs down.

Plant biotechnology of food and feed is another area of consumer interest. If you buy food that comes from overseas, do you ever wonder who oversees the packaging and shipping of those products? Are there really enough inspectors to go around? Consumers worry about the widespread use of sugar in soft drinks. In addition to having your DNA tested, you need to understand how what you eat influences your health at all ages.

Another way consumers can oversee quality control is by forming public interest research groups funded by grant money, private donors, institutions, or the government. You can become a volunteer in nutritional genomics, an ombudsman, a lobbyist, or start your own consumer research interest group.

You can turn a hobby of nutritional genomics or DNA for ancestry and genealogy into a business by affiliating yourself with a university lab which you contract to do testing from your DNA testing clients. There are open doors for consumer involvement depending upon your skills and interests. Nutritional genomics needs public speakers and technical writers to relay to the public what innovations the experts are bringing to healthcare and food systems design.

From running a summer camp for teens interested in nutritional genomics internships or learning experiences to recruiting DNA donors to create a DNA bank or in researching and writing about genomics, there are a variety of doors. Consumers have power in numbers. You can even enter as a venture capitalist with a goal of raising funds even if you have no funds of your own and plenty of determination to learn to ropes.

Don't overlook nutritional genomics for the pet care industry from foods to medicine. Contact the veterinary schools about their research on how foods affect genetic signatures of pets or race horses. Check out the Web site for Research Diets at: http://www.researchdiets.com/.

Research Diets, a New Jersey company since 1984 has formulated more than 6,000 distinct *laboratory* animal diets for research in all areas of biology and related fields at hundreds of pharmaceutical, university, and government laboratories around the world. Nutritional genomics isn't only for humans or laboratory animals. Did you ever think about how your dog or cat could benefit by genetic testing to determine which foods are healthiest?

Talk to your veterinarian to see who is researching how nutraceuticals and better food can help your pet's health, especially when the pet is older. What about nutritional genomics for farm animals or pets? Find out who is doing what kind of nutrition research for better health.

At home-genetic testing needs watchdogs, Web sites, and guidebooks to interpret test results in plain language for those with no science background. Online, you'll find genetic tests for ancestry or for familial (genetic, inherited) disease risks. What helpful suggestions do general consumers with no science background need to consider? What's new in medical marketing is genetic testing online for *predisposition* to diseases—such as breast cancer or blood conditions. Kits usually are sent directly to the consumer who returns a mouthwash or swab DNA sample by mail.

What type of training do healthcare teams need in order to interpret the results of these tests to consumers? Once you receive the results of online genetic testing kits, how do you interpret it? If your personal physician isn't yet trained to interpret the results of online genetic tests, how can you find a healthcare professional that is trained?

If you're more interested in genetic testing for ancestry, do you go to a genealogist or to a geneticist to interpret the results? What if your interest is in genetic testing for disease risks? Do you go to a physician, a nutritionist, a genetics counselor, or a geneticist to find out how certain foods, medicines, dosages, or other products affect your individual genetic expression?

Online firms increasingly market tests that reveal predisposition to diseases. They show risk rather than a sentence that you'll get the disease. Some of these genetic tests offered online show predisposition to breast cancer, blood clotting, or other genetic tendencies. Each day, there's another genetic discovery ranging from varying the dosages of medicines according to one's ethnicity or race mixture to examining the effects of certain foods on certain peoples based on genetic test results. One example would be lactose intolerance—inability to digest milk without symptoms.

Since the human genome code was cracked in the year 2000, scientists have been publishing the results of genetic research, including maps of human, animal, and plant genes. Genetic tests are easy to take. You rub a felt or cotton swab around inside of your mouth and mail it to the testing company according to directions. Your results can be read online. How do you interpret those results?

If you take the results to your doctor, and your physician has never been trained to interpret the results in plain language, you'll need some guidance on how to choose a physician or genetics counselor who has the current training. If the results also were interpreted online, you wouldn't need to visit your physician to get the big picture. So when you take your test, and see your results online, write to your company asking them to also put online samples of how results are interpreted.

Your individual genes will be different from someone else's, but at least you will be able to see in plain language how someone else's tests were interpreted. So far, no detailed interpretations of tests for disease of anonymous individuals are specifically put online for the consumer with little or no science background. Will this day be soon arriving?

What's certain is that DNA tests for predisposition to diseases are affordable and not expensive. Your genetic test results that you take from online testing firms are **not** put into your permanent medical records. That way, private information won't get into the hands of anyone who requests your medical records, like insurance companies and employers chomping at the bit to find out to what you're predisposed.

I like the online approach because it validates your family history. Predictive medicine is the cure of the future. There is a high demand for breast cancer genetic tests through online testing kits.

Personalized medicine and predictive medicine are growing rapidly in revenue and in consumer demand. *If you want to find out what a company's revenues are, begin your research by looking at any company's regulatory filings.* Under the banner "predictive medicine," you can start your search as a consumer. What sells the most? So far, breast cancer genetic tests are popular.

Look for a genetic testing company online that employs its own physicians and genetics counselors who are trained to interpret in plain language to consumers with no science background on how to interpret the results of the specific the types of tests offered. Look for companies that work with doctor's orders and signed informed consent documents for each test.

What you need before you start your research as a consumer of predictive medicine is to be able to reach professionals online. You may even live or work in an area where it's hard to find a doctor. You need to be able to see your results online and be able to reach someone who can interpret those results in plain language so you can follow the diet, dosage, or lifestyle that best suits your individual genetic expression.

It's all about expertise in interpreting the results DNA or other genetic marker tests. Who has the expertise, and how do general consumers find that expert online?

With so few genetic counselors available who are trained (approximately 2,000) how will a genetic counselor explain the results of a genetic test to see how your body responds to various medicine dosages when that counselor is trained to talk about pregnancy?

The jobs for many genetics counselors currently are with firms that work with women that have pregnancy concerns. If you want to research this issue on your own, start with the studies of primary care physicians done by the Center for Disease Control and Prevention.

Focus on the particular studies of primary care physicians' inability to handle the overwhelming demand for genetic testing but only after the genetic tests were advertised in the media. Note that these types of studies are usually restricted to certain parts of the country.

Any good university library or medical school library has articles and studies on their shelves, but few consumers take the time to research studies concerning the demand for genetic testing, particular tests marketed online. Medical marketing focuses more on TV and magazine advertising of drugs rather than marketing online genetic testing kits in popular magazines.

Is there a way consumers can catch up with technology? Yes, online, if the online material is perceived and verified as credible. So what can the consumer with no science background do—get involved in public policy and team up with scientists? That's the first step—empowering yourself by learning to interpret complex DNA test results if only for your individual markers.

You'll need a physician trained to interpret genetic test results and a genetics counselor on your team, but you need this type of team consisting of consumer and professional—online together. No doctor is going to handle a flood of demand for genetic test kit interpretation.

What can you do? You can offer an online company that does nothing but interpret the results and acts as a middle person connecting consumer and physician. What you can do is start that type of online company provided the better mouse trap, that is, the online company that will interpret DNA tests given by other online companies.

Another position the general consumer can take is to seek to regulate the market. You can open a company that validates the online companies. And if you don't want to open a company, you can research and offer information to consumers and to physicians.

What if you are a consumer who only wants a genetic test to find out whether you're predisposed to a specific disease such as breast cancer? According to DNA Direct, located in San Francisco, the company is online and has assembled a dedicated staff of genetic and medical experts.

DNA Direct provides direct-to-consumer personalized genetic testing services that help consumers put their genes in context with their overall health, lifestyle, and environment. With the permission of DNA Direct to reprint, here is what the informational literature of DNA Direct reports:

About DNA Direct

The results of each test are paired with an in-depth Personalized Report that combines an individual's unique test results, lifestyle and health concerns with a practical plan for action. Each report includes scientific research and extensive resources. In addition, customers are encouraged to call or email DNA Direct's genetic experts for further discussion, interpretation and/or resources and information. DNA Direct believes that testing is about empowerment—your body and your health are ultimately your responsibility.

And your genes offer tremendous insight and play a vital role in the personal, medical and lifestyle choices you make. DNA Direct is a privately held company, incorporated in the fall of 2003, located in San Francisco, California. The company is staffed by a group of dedicated individuals and genetic experts committed to building a genetic testing service that empowers health care consumers.

Genetic testing offers information that can help people make informed decisions about medical management and lifestyle choices. In the current healthcare model, not everyone has access to genetic testing for a variety of reasons.

In genetics publishing, this is the era of making the Web pay. Smart foods, DNA-driven ancestry, molecular anthropology, and genealogy-related books reached the general consumer market beginning in 2002. Currently, the human genome, DNA profiling, smart foods, and personalized medicine are big news and big publishing. Online genetic testing with direct-to consumer contact provides an open door to predictive medicine and nutrition research.

As mandated by medical professional societies, genetic tests must often be ordered by a physician and test results are interpreted by a genetic counselor, geneticist, or specialist. In some states, genetic testing must be accompanied by an in-person genetics evaluation and/or genetic counseling appointment.

This approach is limited by the fact that there are only 1,200 medical geneticists and just over 2,000 genetic counselors in the US, most often based in urban areas. The number and type of genetic tests are growing exponentially, and they provide a unique opportunity for consumers to learn more about their health. (Note that the prices of various tests and types of tests mentioned for DNA Direct (below) are how they appeared at the time this book went to press. Please contact the company for any updates in information.)

◆   ◆   ◆

DNA Direct's Solution

DNA Direct provides individuals with access to confidential genetic testing using quality-assured tests from CLIA-certified labs. DNA Direct's Web-based genetic testing service redefines traditional, face-to-face genetic counseling and allows individuals to be proactive in managing their care. **Why test?** People seek genetic testing for a variety of reasons, including medical, social, emotional and financial.

- Knowledge about your genes can help you make better decisions for your health and for your family.

- The results of a test can give you specific information about your unique body—and you could be empowered to take actions that really make changes in your life.

- Your genes combine with other factors to influence your health. To understand what your test results really mean, they need to be interpreted in the context of your overall health, lifestyle, and environment.

- From peace-of-mind to prevention or treatment, genetic information can tailor your healthcare to best suit your needs.

How Testing Works:

DNA Direct's genetic testing services are high quality, confidential and convenient. The company offers genetic tests that are scientifically proven and performed by CLIA-certified labs. As new tests become commercially available, DNA Direct has the ability to evaluate and make them available to consumers. DNA Direct's solution is simple, easy to use and a certified genetic expert is available to answer questions at any point in the decision, testing, results and reporting process (M-F, 9:00 a.m.—5 p.m. PST). Here's how it works:

Step 1: Get Informed

Learn about genetic testing and determine whether a genetic test is right for you. Knowing whether a medical condition has a genetic basis can be the first step in taking action to live a longer, healthier life. The Web site features:

- Information about specific genetic tests

- A Resource Center with information on genetic conditions, basic genetic concepts, and family stories
- "Why Take a Genetic Test?" and other information on testing

Step 2: Purchase a Test Online, Submit a Sample

The test is easy, painless and completely anonymous with DNA Direct's secure ordering process. Once ordered, a test kit is sent to you. Each kit contains:

- A cheek-swab home test kit[1]
- A postage-paid return envelope
- An informed consent form

To test, simply swab the inside of your cheeks with the test kit swabs. Then mail them to the lab in the envelope provided. If you have already had genetic testing, DNA Direct's experts can prepare a Personalized Report using existing test results.

Privacy is of the utmost importance. All personal information is and remains private. Within two business days of purchase, you will receive a genetic test kit in a discreet mailer.

Step 3: View Results & Personalized Report

When the lab result is ready (7-10 days after sample is received), you will receive an email with a password-protected link to your Personalized Report. Simply click on the link, and log in using the secure email and password. The report can be printed, referenced later or shared with others, such as a physician.

Genes are only one piece of the health puzzle. A person's history, lifestyle and other factors also play an important role. The Personalized Report is an essential component to putting your genes in context and giving him or her tools and information to make informed choices. All DNA Direct's genetic tests are accompanied by individually tailored Web reports, which interpret test results in the context of these factors, and explain them in plain English. A Personalized Report includes:

- Lab results and an easy-to-understand explanation of the results.
- Suggestions on how to improve your health and reduce your risk.

---

1.   Some tests require a blood sample. For these, DNA Direct provides simple tools to help locate a local clinic affiliate to have a simple, anonymous blood sample taken.

- What your results mean to your family, how to talk with your family or doctor

- A physician's letter should you wish to consult your doctor

- Links to other resources, further reading and support services.

- Toll-free access to DNA Direct's genetic experts for additional support and education. DNA Direct's certified genetic counselors are available from 9:00 a.m. to 5:00 p.m. PST, Monday-Friday, 1.877.646.0222 or via email at expert@dnadirect.com.

DNA Direct's Commitment to Your Well Being

Genetics is all DNA Direct does. Its dedication means consumers benefit from the latest research and developments in this fast-moving area of science. DNA Direct collects genetic news and scientific updates of interest to our customers. The DNA Direct Web site offers information on basic genetics, diseases and conditions, FAQs, the latest research, and more.

DNA Direct brings its customers the latest news on their health and genetic concerns, and it encourages them to stay up-to-date on the health news and medical research that's most important to them by subscribing to DNA Direct's News Alerts (no personal information, including email addresses is ever shared). For additional information about DNA Direct, services and support, call 1-877-646-0222.

DNA Direct leverages the Internet to offer personalized genetic tests to help consumers make more informed healthcare choices. DNA Direct's confidential genetic testing offers consumers unparalleled access and insight with personalized reports and genetic expert support.

According to DNA Direct's press release of February 9, 2005, the Internet has clearly become a valued resource for consumers seeking healthcare information. Today, DNA Direct is helping people go one step further by providing individuals with unparalleled access to confidential genetic testing, insight into their personal genetic make-up, expert genetic support and links to resources that can help them lead longer, healthier lives.

As a direct-to-consumer genetic testing company, DNA Direct offers consumers an unprecedented array of genetic tests and pairs each test result with a comprehensive, personalized interpretation. The result is a highly confidential means for people to take a more active role in their health and well being.

"Genetic testing can help us understand who we are and empowers an individual to make informed decisions about health management," says Katherine

Rauen, MD, Ph.D, DNA Direct's Medical Director. "With just over 2,000 genetic counselors nationwide and even fewer medical geneticists, most people don't have access to genetic testing. DNA Direct is bridging this gap to provide people with a resource to better understand, evaluate and, if they choose, work with their physicians to better manage their health and healthcare decisions."

"DNA Direct provides access to those genetic tests where knowing about your genes can make a big difference, such as when planning a family, selecting a form of birth control or starting hormone replacement therapy," said Ryan Phelan, Founder and CEO, DNA Direct. "It's important to keep in mind that genes are not the sole factor in determining an individual's destiny—family history, lifestyle and environment all play an integral part."

The results of a genetic test can help confirm or rule out a suspected genetic condition or help determine an individual's risk of developing or passing on a genetic disorder.

- Studies estimate that 60,000 to 200,000 people die each year from blood clots. At the high end, this disease kills more people than breast cancer, car accidents and AIDS combined. And 1 in 20 Americans carry a gene, factor V Leiden, which can increase the risk for dangerous blood clots when combined with medical treatments (hormone replacement therapy, birth control pills) or other factors (obesity, smoking, long-haul plane flights). When you know you have genetic propensity for blood clots, you can take action to minimize your risk. (DNA Direct Test at the time this book went to press): Thrombophilia; cost: $380)

- About 35 million people in the U.S.—as many as 1 in 4 people of Irish descent, and 1 in 10 Caucasians—are at risk for a hereditary iron overload disorder that causes a wide variety of symptoms, including chronic fatigue, weakness, joint pain and arthritis. If undetected, iron overload can lead to serious problems, including diabetes, liver and heart disease. But with early detection, effective treatment can stop the progression and even reverse some of the symptoms. (DNA Direct Test: Hemochromatosis; cost at Direct DNA (at the time this book went to press): $199.25)

- About 116 million people worldwide—and up to 1 in 10 Americans—are Alpha-1 carriers. Alpha-1 antitrypsin deficiency is one of the most common genetic disorders worldwide. It is often misdiagnosed, most often as asthma. Early diagnosis can help people at risk take steps to prevent lung and liver disease. A simple genetic test is available for alpha-1 antitrypsin deficiency. (DNA

Direct Test: Alpha-1 Antitrypsin Deficiency; cost at Direct DNA (at the time this book went to press): $330).

DNA Direct currently offers the following genetic tests:

- **Chronic Lung/Liver Disease** (Alpha1-Antitrypsin)
- **Cystic Fibrosis** (CFTR)
- **Hereditary Iron Overload** (Hemochromatosis, HFE)
- **Inherited Blood Clotting Disorders** (Factor V Leiden and Prothrombin)
- **Infertility Panel** (Fragile—X, Cystic Fibrosis, Thrombophilia, Hemochromatosis, Chromosome Analysis, Y Chromosome Deletion)

Ask about DNA Direct's tests for inherited cancer susceptibility. All prices include a Personalized Report that **interprets results** and offers personalized suggestions for lowering risk, and making well-informed decisions about healthcare. Each report also includes information about putting together a healthcare team, and how to approach sharing information with family members and your physician. Due to confidentiality considerations, DNA Direct does not process insurance claims but does provide information and documentation should you choose to submit an insurance claim on your own.

About DNA Direct

San Francisco-based DNA Direct is a personalized genetic testing company focused on consumer education, empowerment and support. With a promise of providing "Your Genes in Context," DNA Direct's mission is to empower individuals with insight into their genetic make-up, including risk factors, preventive measures and action-oriented information to reduce personal risk, coupled with one-on-one support from DNA Direct's genetic experts. All of DNA Direct's services are completely confidential. For more information, go to the Web site at: http://www.dnadirect.com.

Personalized Genetic Tests Offered

The results of a genetic test can help confirm or rule out a suspected genetic condition or help determine an individual's risk of developing or passing on a genetic disorder. Once a genetic condition is known, preventative and/or treatment choices can often be made. All DNA Direct tests are selected to help people make better health care and lifestyle decisions. DNA Direct currently offers the following genetic tests:

- **Chronic Lung/Liver Disease** (Alpha1-Antitrypsin)
- **Cystic Fibrosis** (CFTR)
- **Hereditary Iron Overload** (Hemochromatosis, HFE)
- **Inherited Blood Clotting Disorders** (Factor V Leiden and Prothrombin)
- **Infertility Panel** (Fragile—X, Cystic Fibrosis, Thrombophilia, Hemochromatosis, Chromosome Analysis, Y Chromosome Deletion)

All prices include a Personalized Report that interprets results and offers personalized suggestions for lowering risk, and making well-informed healthcare decisions. Each report also includes information about putting together a healthcare team, and sharing information with family members and your physician. Due to confidentiality considerations, DNA Direct does not process insurance claims but does provide information and documentation should individuals choose to submit insurance claims on their own.

TEST: INHERITED BLOOD CLOTTING DISORDERS (THROMBOPHILIA)

More than 19 million Americans carry a gene for thrombophilia. If you are one of them, you can take action to prevent dangerous blood clots and live a healthier life. Studies estimate that 60,000 to 200,000 people die each year from blood clots.

At the high end, this disease kills more people than breast cancer, car accidents and AIDS combined. And 1 in 20 Americans carry the gene, factor V Leiden, which can increase the risk for dangerous blood clots when combined with medical treatments (hormone replacement therapy, birth control pills) or other factors (obesity, smoking, long-haul plane flights). When you know you have genetic propensity for blood clots, you can take action to minimize your risk.

Quality Lab Analysis:	DNA analysis of the two most common mutations in the factor V and prothrombin genes by a CLIA-certified laboratory.
Home Test Kit:	Cheek Swab

Test Process:	Order a test online and receive a test kit in the mail. Use the pain-less cheek swab in the privacy of your home and mail it to our lab in the postage-paid envelope. When the results are ready, we notify you by email. Log on to your secure, password protected account to get your results and Personalized Report online.
Personalized Report:	Explains test results and interprets your genes in context, consid-ering age, health, lifestyle, family concerns, preventive steps, resources and much more.
Expert Support:	Genetics experts are available to answer questions and provide support (toll-free 877-646-0222 or expert@dnadirect.com)
Price:	$380

TEST: IRON OVERLOAD (HEMOCHROMATOSIS)

Hemochromatosis is an iron overload disorder that can effectively be prevented or treated—but it is often undiagnosed or misdiagnosed. About 35 million peo-ple in the U.S.—as many as 1 in 4 people of Irish descent, and 1 in 10 Cauca-sians—are at risk for a hereditary iron overload disorder that causes a wide variety of symptoms, including chronic fatigue, weakness, joint pain and arthritis. If undetected, iron overload can lead to serious problems, including diabetes, liver and heart disease. But with early detection, effective treatment can stop the pro-gression and even reverse some of the symptoms.

Quality Lab Analysis:	DNA analysis of the two most common mutations in the HFE gene by a CLIA-certified laboratory.
Home Test Kit:	Cheek Swab
Test Process:	Order a test online and receive a test kit in the mail. Use the pain-less cheek swab in the privacy of your home and mail it to our lab in the postage-paid envelope. When the results are ready, we notify you by email. Log on to your secure, password protected account to get your results and Personalized Report online.
Personalized Report:	Explains test results and interprets your genes in context, consid-ering age, health, lifestyle, family history, preventive steps, resources and much more.

| Expert Support: | Genetics experts are available to answer questions and provide support (toll-free 877-646-0222 or expert@ dnadirect.com) |
| Price: | $199.25 |

TEST: CHRONIC LUNG/LIVER DISEASE (ALPHA1-ANTITRYPSIN)

Alpha-1 antitrypsin deficiency is one of the most common genetic disorders worldwide. It is often misdiagnosed, most often as asthma. In early stages it can cause breathing difficulties, fatigue, and weakness, and eventually it can lead to chronic obstructive lung disease (COPD), emphysema, and liver failure. Early diagnosis can help people at risk take steps to prevent lung and liver disease. About 116 million people worldwide—and up to 1 in 10 Americans—are Alpha-1 carriers.

Quality Lab Analysis:	DNA analysis of the two most common mutations in the Alpha-1 gene by a CLIA-certified laboratory.
Home Test Kit:	Cheek Swab
Test Process:	Order a test online and receive a test kit in the mail. Use the painless cheek swab in the privacy of your home and mail it to our lab in the postage-paid envelope. When the results are ready, we notify you by email. Log on to your secure, password protected account to get your results and Personalized Report online.
Personalized Report:	Explains test results and interprets your genes in context, considering age, health, lifestyle, family history, preventive steps, resources and much more.
Expert Support:	Genetics experts are available to answer questions and provide support (toll-free 877-646-0222 or expert@ dnadirect.com)
Price:	$330

PANEL TEST: INFERTILITY

Infertility Panel:

Tests Included:	Fragile—X, Cystic Fibrosis, Thrombophilia, Hemochromatosis, Chromosome Analysis, Y Chromosome Deletion
Home Test Kit:	Blood sample
Test Process:	Order a test online and receive a test kit in the mail. Visit a nearby clinic affiliate to have a simple, anonymous blood sample taken. Mail your informed consent in the postage-paid envelope to DNA Direct. When the results are ready, we notify you by email. Log on to your secure, password protected account to get your results and Personalized Report online.
Personalized Report:	Explains test results and interprets your genes in context, considering age, health, lifestyle, family concerns, preventive steps, resources and much more.
Expert Support:	Genetics experts are available to answer questions and provide support (toll-free 877-646-0222 or expert@ dnadirect.com)
Price:	male panel $1248.25, female panel $1,191.50

- Prices subject to change without further notice

◆   ◆   ◆

Responding to Food or Medicine—What Are the Debates?

Some DNA testing companies that are online test for reactions to medicines or foods, such as the speed at which your body metabolizes anesthetic. Can you trust what you read online when so many unscreened and diverse opinions are there? How do you find an expert willing to answer specific questions?

Unless you're a member of credible media with a letter of assignment from your editor, how do you know the person responding is giving you a responsible answer? Should you attend scientific conventions as a way of getting your questions answered? Who has the time and willingness to answer your questions, and is the person really an expert in the branch of science you need?

Online you'll find numerous companies marketing various DNA tests or kits. Some of these genetic tests are to find out how your body reacts to various dosages of drugs or even foods and skin products. How do you tailor your medicines, foods, exercise, activities, cosmetics, anesthetics, dosages, or lifestyles to your genetic signature?

Can you find out by genetic tests which type of dental anesthesia you can tolerate and which you're type makes you feel jittery or convulsive? What about tests to find out how your hair tint affects your heart beat? What kinds of tests are out there?

You'll need a consumer's guide to genetic testing kits. Research the various companies online and the studies that include side effects of whatever product or medicine you think you might have to use. Your goal is to safely tailor your environment and lifestyle to your genetic expression or signature. Ask questions of experts on the specific issue you want to understand.

Consumer's Guide to Genetic Testing

Your DNA, including your ancient ancestry and ethnicity has a lot to do with how your body responds to food, medicine, illness, exercise, and lifestyle, but just how much? And how do you know which DNA kits and gene testing are reliable and recognized?

Learning about DNA to understand and improve your health is now interactive and available to the average consumer, not limited to students and teachers, but to anyone else. In the last few years genealogy buffs, parents, and anyone interested in DNA without a science background took an interest in DNA tests rests that reveal deep maternal and paternal ancestry.

Currently consumers with little or no science background are interested in learning about drug metabolism—pharmacogenetics. Referring to the whole human genome that science related to linking pharmacy with genetics is called pharmacogenomics.

How your body metabolizes medicine is as important as how your body metabolizes food. Nutrigenomics is about how your genes respond to food and how to tailor what you eat to your DNA. Consumer DNA interest ranges from forensics and anthropology to nutrition, caregiving, family scrapbooking and healthcare knowledge.

Nurses are becoming more interested in DNA. The DNA consumer revolution began when media broadcasts revealed to the public that fast computers had revealed the human gene code. Once more TV opened doors. Suddenly, a gap between science and consumers had to be bridged by available interactive education.

A proliferation of products relating to DNA emerged. The internet shows DNA summer day camps for students and teachers. DNA testing companies and books emerged geared to the average consumer. Genealogists tried to interpret DNA for ancestry. People left other non-science-related businesses to open up DNA testing companies for ancestry research, contracting out to university research laboratories to do the DNA testing. Again, opportunities opened doors to the public.

Nutrigenomics product marketers sought those who wanted a diet tailored to their genetic signature. Pharmacogenetics reports customized medicines in order to prevent adverse drug reactions. Pharmacogenomics studies the entire genome in relation to chemicals and drugs, whereas pharmacogenetics researches specific genes and markers to look for adverse drug reactions for individual clients or patients. Finally, DNA testing products emerged offering to tailor skin care products such as creams and cosmetics to your individual genetic signature.

If you've had an interest in learning about how to interpret your DNA test results for ancestry, you now can see the links to understanding how to tailor your food, lifestyle, exercise, medicines, supplements, and skin care products—in fact numerous environmental chemicals—to your genetic expression. It's not only about food anymore or ancestry alone, or medicine.

DNA testing also is about kits sent to you directly or to your physician. It's about tailoring to your DNA skin products, cosmetics and anything you put into or on your body that gets absorbed. It's about what chemicals are in your water and home-grown vegetables.

No science background? Don't worry. There's a DNA summer camp near you, or an educational experience in learning about DNA now available to the average consumer. Educators, scientists, and multimedia producers have teamed up to teach you the wonders of DNA, your genes and your lifestyle.

What's left? Physicians and genetic research scientists need to talk more to each other because most family doctors don't have time to read the proliferation of publications reporting new advances in genetics or other areas of science that directly affect consumers. It looks like it's the consumer's job to bring people together through the media and through consumer's watchdog organizations, professional associations, and support groups. Key words: action and public education about DNA through multimedia and consumer involvement. I highly recommend the DNA Interactive Web site at: http://www.dnalc.org/.

Consumers need to know more about how to interpret DNA test results for whatever purpose they seek—tailoring diets or drugs, skin care products, or seeking out ancient family history or ancestral lineages. The science is new enough to have many more applications on the horizon that consumers can digest in the future. What can the average consumer with no science background learn about applications of DNA testing currently? Start with the publications and the interactive DNA learning sites.

You'll soon become familiar with the DNA terminology. The goal is to bridge the gap between science and the consumer. How do you narrow the gap between ethnobotany, genetics, and health care practices when physicians, geneticists, biochemists, medical anthropologists, and ethnobotanists may not share information easily with one another and with the public because they move in different circles and read different scientific journals? You'll have to invite your busy family doctor to join you in creating consumer groups.

It'll work fine. Doctors and scientists usually are found conversing together at parties. You, as the media, may have to get them talking more during working hours at a time when they have fewer hours available for networking.

The triangle of journalist-scientist/dietician-physician now includes the consumer. If you have children, bring them into the fold. There are now wonderful DNA summer camps. So include your children's teachers. Learning about DNA as a consumer might make you wish you had majored in genetics. Link your beginning self-taught DNA studies to your special field of interest such as your healthcare or your ancestry.

For history buffs, there's always molecular genealogy for family history. History buffs can follow population genetics. Anthropology enthusiasts can read about archaeogenetics. Bring archaeology and DNA together.

Nutrigenomics links DNA research to nutrition for the diet-conscious. Pharmacogenetics helps you to tailor specific medicines to your genes. DNA gets into all walks of life and work. Find out what field you need to research first—nutrition, pharmacy, genealogy, anthropology, or heathcare. Read a book about discoveries or research for beginners on DNA and nutrition related to understanding your particular area of interest. The following are some activities to consider:

- Discoveries are published monthly in recognized scientific journals found in local medical school libraries open to the public. Only a few consumers ever look at them, and still fewer physicians. Conduct guided tours of university libraries aimed at members of the press, parents, teachers, students, librarians, nurses, dental assistants, publicists, and freelance writers' groups.

- Doctors are busy with so many patients and paperwork or bureaucracy. Consumers may not know information is accessible to them. And few can keep up with the proliferation of material in science publications. Create support groups at library conference rooms that bridge the gap between science and the consumer.

- For information, resources, the research network, and references on pharmacogenetics (education) see the Pharmacogenetics and Pharmacogenomics Knowledge Base Web site at: https://preview.pharmgkb.org/resources/education.jsp. As far as education, the Web site features links and articles on the following subjects: What is Pharmacogenetics? Asthma Case Study, CYP2D6 Case Study, The National Institutes of General Medical Sciences (NIGMS), Medicines For You, Minority Pharmacogenomics, The Importance of Genetic Variation in Drug Development, Publications, and News Clippings.

- Click on the Dolan DNA Learning Center at: http://www.dnalc.org/. The Dolan DNA Learning Center at Cold Spring Harbor is entirely devoted to public genetics education. The gene almanac is an online resource that provides timely information about genes in education. The Dolan DNA Learning Center is the world's first science museum and educational facility promoting DNA literacy.

- Dolan's Saturday DNA program is designed to offer children, teens and adults the opportunity to perform hands-on DNA experiments and learn about the latest developments in the biological sciences. Promote hands-on activities in science for groups of all ages—students to senior citizens for life-long learning projects.

- If you're interested in student "DNA Camps" see the Web site at: http://www.dnalc.org/programs/workshops.html. Student summer day camps have fun with DNA and enzymes and study DNA science or genetic biology. Students and high-school teachers can participate. There are a lot of ways to become involved in learning more on these topics. I wish there were DNA day camps for senior citizens newly retired with time free at last, or for parents, children, and teachers to participate and learn together.

The student summer day camp workshops feature such wonderful learning experiences as the genomic biology and PCR workshop. This new workshop is based on lab and computer technology developed at the DNALC in the past year. The workshop focuses on the use of the polymerase chain reaction (PCR) to analyze the genetic complement (genome) of humans and plants. DNA educational centers bridge gaps between scientists and communicators.

Many physicians have not yet been trained in nutritional genomics or in pharmacogenetics—how to correctly interpret a DNA test for consumers. Who advises consumers how to tailor their food or drugs to their genes in ways that consumers can immediately use? Who instructs them how to make time capsules out of their ancestry from DNA reports?

For the time being, it's the bioscience journalist who acts as a communicator, the liaison, the publicist, the broadcaster, the bearer of news, the turner of complex terms into plain language, the reporter and the publisher, showing consumers, physicians, and scientists how to bridge the gap between science and healthcare.

Who acts as the middle person between genetics and medicine or between nutrition and healthcare? Who bridges the gap between the dietician and the geneticist? For now, it's the media, the science writer writing for the mass media or an audience of general readers—consumers like you and I. Who should join the science media team? Check out consumer watchdog groups, concerned physicians, genetics researchers—scientists, DNA testing companies, and bioscience publishers.

Instead of worrying about physician apathy or consumers turning to alternative medicine, let's turn to scientific knowledge available to all consumers if you know where to look and what is accessible. If you want to take charge over how your body responds to food or medicine or lifestyle changes, you need to take control by finding out how your genes respond to what you put into your body from what you eat to the drugs you take to the chemicals in your environment.

Has a local or national newspaper reported on rocket fuel or other specific chemicals in your water supply that went into your home-grown vegetables that made your thyroid go wild, find out what research is being done on the situation. Or if your body responds to various foods in certain ways or various drugs in other ways, you can take control by learning what new advances are available to you.

Check out what is credible and what works for you. Minorities may have genes that respond differently to various dosages of medicines. Check out the Web site for research on minority pharmacogenetics at: <http://www.sph.uth.tmc.edu:8057/gdr/default.htm>. The Minority Pharmacogenetics website is devoted to issues of minorities, populations and pharmacogenomics.

Have you ever met a doctor who keeps up with all the latest advances? Who has time? Consumers do. Look at the breakthroughs in the journals published monthly. Why worry that medical discoveries aren't being delivered fast enough to patients or clients if you can see what's happening in the journals?

Consumers need to form watchdog groups and to link up with the media. You need to become involved in accessing scientific pioneers. As a journalist, my job is to convey information to the public to bridge the communication gap. As a consumer, your job is to take care of your body.

Nobody should walk in medical or nutritional ignorance when the information you might need "is out there." You don't need any science degree or license to read public information. Let's all bridge the communication gap between consumers, scientists, and physicians.

Consumers want applied knowledge. Here's where to start. On the Web, look at: http://www.nigms.nih.gov/funding/medforyou.html. It's the page for The National Institutes of General Medical Sciences (NIGMS). It's the home page for the National Institute of General Medical Sciences, a component of the National Institutes of Health, the principle biomedical research agency of the United States Government. "NIGMS supports basic biomedical research that is not targeted to specific diseases, but that increases understanding of life processes and lays the foundation for advances in disease diagnosis, treatment, and prevention," according to the Pharmacogenetics and Pharmactogenomics Knowledge Base at: http://www.nigms.nih.gov/funding/medforyou.html.

If your doctor hasn't the time to take advantage of current treatment findings, you as a consumer can read what your physician may not get to read for a while. Consumers can help to bridge the gap between research and conventional medicine by connecting with the media with scientists as a bridge carrying the voice of the consumer.

Learn to interpret scientific findings in plain language by first talking to librarians who will direct you to summaries and abstracts of scientific journal articles. You might debate the issue of how valuable are nutrition applications from genetic test results. What can be applied to real-life situations? Can you list the issues and controversies surrounding tailoring your food to your genetic signatures? All this information falls under the umbrella of personalized medicine. Included are subjects such as infant gender selection, and customized food and medicines based on predictive medicine. Can we rely on genetic tests at this stage? Genetic testing is still in its infancy. Those are some of the controversies.

What kind of personalized medicine can consumers find today regarding genetic testing? How many ways can you use DNA tests? Tailoring your food, customizing your medicines by avoiding adverse drug reactions, looking at your ancient ancestry? What are the relationships between what you eat and the scientific study of molecular genetics? What if the findings change frequently? How do you keep up with the information?

How many ways can you market DNA tests? For what purposes in the field of nutrition can you use DNA tests? Who will review the products? Who is writing the guides to genetic testing kits sold directly to the public? How does the informational literature differ from guides sold only to healthcare professionals?

Personalized Medicine from DNA Testing Companies

Who regulates doctors' services? Are DNA test kits doctor's services? Or are they medical devices? What will consumers pay to have their healthcare and nutrition tailored to their individual genetic signatures? Most want tests to be affordable and available to everyone. What's more important? Testing some genes to see how fast your body metabolizes anesthesia or other drugs? Or testing certain genes to see how your body uses certain foods or vitamins and minerals?

The FDA regulates medical devices, not physician's services. Where does a DNA kit sent directly to consumers fit into a definition? Scientists and physicians study haplotypes when they map complex-disease genes. Genetic researchers look at the abundance of single-nucleotide polymorphisms (SNPs). They use terms such as "single-locus analyses."

Consumers want those terms translated into plain language by bioscience communicators, since most scientists and physicians are too busy to continuously write about genes for the public. That's why public education programs about DNA exist, including the summer day camps for students and teachers. We need the training programs and camps also for parents—for entire families from great grandma and pa to elementary school children and teens.

When it comes to studying how your genes respond to food or drugs, scientists avoid analyses techniques with limited power and instead focus on economical alternatives to molecular-haplotyping methods. So you, as a consumer, presumably with little or no science background, are in a position to learn about your own genes and about DNA in general.

You can start with some of the DNA public education learning programs open to anyone. Since the gene hunters began to explore the entire human genome, they opened a door to the public for knowledge accessible to all. At first consumers were interested in learning how to interpret their DNA test for ancestry and family history. Next, consumers wanted to know how to tailor their drugs and food to their genes—their genetic expression. Finally, consumers found they could customize skin care products to their DNA reports as well.

Consumers ask important questions. What's waiting for you in a DNA kit that will be valuable to your health? How will you understand and apply the scientific reports to your daily lifestyle? How do you find out whether the various DNA testing companies are credible and recognized by which group?

Who are the watchdogs here? Who are the experts? What do you do with the information you receive after a DNA test? Should you test for deep ancestry, adverse response to drugs, or tailoring your food to your DNA? How do you apply the information in a practical way?

Should the consumer only deal with companies that sell their DNA test kits to physicians and similar healthcare professions such as dieticians and genetics counselors? Or should the average consumer buy a DNA testing kit directly from a company that also markets to consumers, bypassing physicians? What do you think as a consumer? Which stance are you taking? For resources and articles, see the Web site at: http://syndromexmenu.tripod.com.

What happens when a DNA testing company sells its DNA tests or kits to companies that turn around and sell personalized nutritional or cosmetics products so that consumers can buy skin products or nutritional supplements customized to their genetic signatures? Is this good for consumers? Interpretation of the tests is tricky. Results can have a lot more than one interpretation, even for physicians and scientists. So how does the consumer learn to screen the screeners? Who watches the watchers?

Should a company tell consumers which specific genes are tested? Some companies do and others don't. How do you know whether the dose of vitamins you take is beneficial or harmful? Do you need to cut back or add more? What can DNA testing do for you, the consumer, presumably starting with no science background?

Some types of genetic test kits are sold directly to the public, and others are marketed only to physicians and similar healthcare professionals. From the consumer's point of view, there is always the question of whether the tests are needed and if they are, how accurate and valuable are the tests, and who is trained and experienced enough to interpret the answers?

If you're going to take a DNA test, it could be for ancestry, for nutrition planning, or to see whether any prescribed or over-the-counter drug, chemical, supplement, nutraceutical, food, or herb you take will have adverse effects on your body. For years you could test for allergies to some substances and foods, some chemicals in the environment, but now there's genetic testing.

Specific genes are tested for risk or reaction. The type of consumer most likely to order a genetic test for drug response or a "pharmacogenetic test" would be an individual with medical conditions taking several drugs and concerned how his or her body handled the mix of medicines, food, and lifestyle. Each person has his or her own genetic signature.

You rinse your mouth with a type of mouthwash and send the contents in a small tube to a laboratory, hospital, office, or company to be analyzed. Or you swab the inside of your cheek with a felt tip and send the swab to a hospital or genetic testing company so your DNA—specific genetic markers—can be analyzed.

In a few weeks, you get a report. The genetic testing company looks at specific genes and markers. If you're concerned about drugs, you want to know how slowly your body is breaking down any of the drugs you take or might take in the future.

You don't want to gulp down a prescription or over-the-counter drug and have it build up in your body to the point you land in the emergency room of a hospital. The whole point of a genetic test for adverse drug reactions is to alert your physician to adjust the dosage of your medicine or change the type of medicine.

Here is what one nutrition and genomics debate is about: on one side, the consumer sees the physician and scientist diagnosing rare diseases by looking at particular genes. On the other, the consumer wants information on how genes work.

Firms that sell gene tests directly to consumers need to fill an education gap. Certain tests can be sold directly to consumers, such as DNA testing for ancestry, genealogy, family, oral history, DNA matches, and surname projects where people with the same or similar last names are matched by DNA to see whether there's a relationship in former times.

What DNA testing companies can do for the consumer is to widely teach the consumer about population genetics—the peopling of the world. How about for disease? Genetic disease specialists have been in charge of this new science.

Lately, companies that test DNA now market directly to consumers as well as to their physicians. Here's a chance to educate consumers as well as physicians in everything they need to know about their genes. Physicians want to know how to interpret DNA tests for disease markers.

Consumers want this information directly. So there needs to be a level for education for both physician and consumer.

If a DNA testing firm markets directly to the consumer, the test should be interpreted for the consumer and the physician. Consumers are paying to learn what medications to avoid. Allergists usually told people what foods to avoid. What consumers want is to know what foods, vitamins, minerals, supplements, skin creams, herbs, medicines, and other nutraceuticals will work best with their individual genetic signatures. Who will teach them?

If the physician has only a few minutes to consult with each patient, who else has the time? Either the DNA testing companies must educate the consumer, or the consumer as an autodidact, must teach himself from reliable sources.

Today anyone with a genealogy hobby an open a DNA testing company and contract out to a laboratory in a university to test DNA for clients. When it comes to test DNA for diseases or drug reactions, it's different than sending a printout regarding the client's ancient general ancestry such as the results of a DNA test for mtDNA (matrilineal ancestry) or Y-chromosome (patrilineal ancestry) in the deep past. Those tests are general and would be of interest to people matching ancestors or learning about population genetics an ancient migrations.

When it comes to tailoring food or drugs to your genotype, how far can DNA testing companies bypass the genetic disease specialists and market directly to the consumer? The answer is as far as it takes to teach the consumer about his or her own genetic expression.

When you look for a DNA testing company, ask yourself whether the company diagnoses diseases? Does the company help you choose your medicines, food, or cosmetics according to your genetic signature? Or does the company work with your physician and you. Does the company pass you over entirely and only send the results to your personal physician?

Look at the marketing efforts of the company. Investigate gene research for yourself by the many articles available online and in the medical libraries and popular magazines that go to physicians. If you buy a test, is it affordable? Do you need the particular DNA test?

If one of your relatives has a specific condition you might have inherited that will show symptoms when you reach a certain age or presently, you need to know what you can do to delay or prevent the situation. You need to know that the results of DNA testing are for a particular purpose, such as testing adverse reactions of your body to certain prescription drugs. Find out the value of the tests from reliable sources. If you start with your personal physician, make sure he or she can correctly interpret a genetics test. Some physicians can't because they were never trained to do so.

Consult the various professional associations for referrals to genetic disease specialists rather than rely on a generalist when it comes to interpreting your test while you learn how to interpret your tests yourself. The purpose is to make sure your physician's interpretation and your interpretation agree. If you have any doubt, you need more information and a second opinion.

What you want to avoid is confusion. Are the tests available today reliable? Find out from several opinions of specialists. To reach these specialists, the professional associations for the various genetic disease specialists would be of help as would the publications.

You can talk to the research labs at universities specializing in genetic testing. The institutes are online and have their own Web sites.

Talk to federal health officials about what's on the consumer market in your country and in other countries. Some people send their DNA swabs to companies and/or labs in other countries. Currently genetic tests are sold without a special 'watch' organization that reviews them.

Read some publications put out by the U.S. Food and Drug Administration (FDA). The FDA wants consumers to become more involved in their own food safety and security monitoring.

Keep a folder on DNA testing company marketing claims and check them out. Think of all the allergy warnings and patch tests on hair products.

Should certain foods such as peanuts and shellfish also have allergy warnings? What about foods that allergists frequently report as common allergens—such as corn, wheat, milk, and eggs?

GeneLink, Inc.

Companies can tell you which mix of vitamins works best or what food to eat based on genetic testing and/or health questionnaires. For example, check out GeneLink Inc., New Jersey. Their Web site is at: http://www.bankdna.com/breakthrough_profiling.html.

According to Multex, an investments site at: http://biz.yahoo.com/p/g/gnlk.ob.html, "GeneLink Inc. is a bioscience company that offers the safe collection and preservation of a family's DNA material for later use by the family to identify and potentially prevent inherited diseases. GeneLink has created a new methodology for single nucleotide polymorphisms (SNPs)-based on genetic profiling. The Company plans to license these proprietary assessments to companies that manufacture or market to the nutraceutical, personal care, skin care and weight-loss industries.

GeneLink's operations can be divided into two segments, the biosciences business, which includes three SNP-based, proprietary genetic indicator tests, and DNA Banking, which involves the use of its proprietary DNA Collection Kit." Contact GeneLink at: 100 S. Thurlow Street, Margate, NJ 08402. See the Web site at: http://biz.yahoo.com/p/g/gnlk.ob.html.

GeneLink also offers gene testing for skin care products. According to a March 6, 2003 media release posted at GeneLink's "In the News" Web page at:

http://www.bankdna.com/news_articles/03_06_03.html,   GeneLink,   Inc.
(OTCBB:GNLK) "entered into a collaborative agreement with DNAPrint
Genomics, Inc. (OTCBB:DNAP) whereby the companies will combine certain
scientific and intellectual property resources to develop and market "next generation" genetic profile tests to the $100 Billion plus personal care and cosmetics
industry. Further details were not disclosed.

"GeneLink invented the first genetically-designed patentable DNA test for
customized skin-care products, and DNAPrint brings its ultra-high throughput
genotype capability and ADMIXMAP platform to the partnership. The companies anticipate screening millions of candidate markers to broaden proprietary
product offerings.

"Tests are designed to assess genetic risks for certain skin and nutritional deficiencies and provide a basis for recommending formulations that have been specifically designed to compensate for these deficiencies."

Check out GeneLink's test which tells clients which mix of vitamins is appropriate for an individual's genes without getting an adverse reaction from the vitamin combination. Still, you need to do your homework on the usefulness of the
tests or the claims. Perhaps you need to deal with a company in another country.

Sciona Ltd.

Sciona Ltd. in England gives nutritional advice based on your DNA and a questionnaire related to your health. *The company sells tests only through doctors
and dieticians.* How do you know which defect is associated with any specific
gene when the gene is defective? With so many interpretations, consumers can
become confused from test results. Sometimes scientists in various companies
don't know which results are accurate predictions. That's why consumer watchdog groups are necessary.

The only problem is that the average consumer usually can't afford to hire
genetics counselors unless they have a specific genetic disease. If you have a
reduced ability to process something, it's not a disease, but unless you take action,
your body could suffer in other ways resulting from the reduced ability to process
an essential nutrient from your diet that your body needs to work with other processes. It's like a chain reaction.

That's why DNA testing is helpful. At the same time, you can't assume some
people need more of one vitamin just because their body processes a nutrient at a
reduced rate. The science is still very new. A lot of data is still in the works. You
don't know whether certain genetic profiles need special diets. Consumers want
to see rare clinical data. Consumers most of all want to know the value of what

the DNA tests predict. And no one wants to take a test and then worry for a decade.

What consumers want are not only tests of prescription drugs and food as to whether adverse reactions happen with individuals based on their genetic testing, but personalized anti-aging formulas, cosmetics, creams, and other products customized to the individual's genetic markers are needed.

These tests must be reliable, consumers say. Feedback is helpful. Customer reviews of the companies are needed. Who will publish customer reviews of the products and the DNA testing firms? These consumer reviews could also include input from scientists and physicians. Physicians should take the DNA testing themselves after they are properly trained to interpret the tests before looking at their patient's results.

Nutritionists and dieticians show concern that medical schools only give very brief and shallow courses in nutrition to graduating physicians. What about a course in interpreting genetics tests? Will this be left to naturopaths and homeopaths? Or can medical schools include courses in DNA test interpretation to physicians other than genetic disease specialists? Healthcare consumers should ask for DNA testing from their HMOs before taking prescribed medicines. Will insurance companies pay for testing?

Look at the various DNA testing companies. Also look at health screening companies. One would be HealthcheckUSA, San Antonio, Texas for example, sells a mail-order test for iron buildup in the blood known as hereditary hemochromatosis. Results go to the consumer. If you need a test for cystic fibrosis or a blood clotting disorder known as factor V Leiden, check out this company. Their Web site is at: http://www.healthcheckusa.com/media.html, or you can write to them at: **HealthcheckUSA,** 8700 Crownhill Rd., Suite 110, San Antonio, TX 78209.

Practicing physicians started HealthCheck USA in 1987 to provide health awareness screening to customers throughout the USA. The tests provided to their customers are the same as those ordered by physicians across the country. Many physicians refer their patients to Healthcheck USA. Since 1987, Health-Check USA has provided over 500,000 health awareness screening tests to satisfied customers nationwide.

The company is associated with the country's major fully accredited medical reference laboratories, to ensure quality, accurate test results. HealthcheckUSA has partnered with Virtual Medical Group, Inc., to offer physician interpretation of results. According to HealthcheckUSA's Web site, "You can have your results reviewed and interpreted by a Board Certified Physician. By selecting the "Physician Interpretation of Results" option, you will be mailed instructions with the hard copy of your results. These instructions will give you a toll free number along with your username and password to access your interpretation 72 hours after your blood draw. This process is completely confidential, private, and secure."

Here the consumer has the best of both worlds. What tests are provided? Check out the list of tests provided at the Web site: http://www. healthcheckusa.com/testsweoffer.php.

When any company does health screening, find out whether it is DNA testing, blood testing, comprehensive tests, or whether you are sent test kits such as for colon cancer screening, prothrombin (factor KII) DNA test, cystic fibrosis (DNA test), Factor V R2 (DNA test) or other. Are the results sent back to you directly as a consumer? Or do you purchase additional services such as a physician's interpretation of the results?

What consumers want are genetic tests for metabolism and health. Doctors used genetic testing when patients were concerned about diagnosing inherited diseases. Today, the general consumer of healthcare and healthcare alternative medicine wants genetic testing for general healthcare in the absence of a specific disease. Consumers want to know how to handle the risks they might have inherited to delay or prevent what happened to their grandparents. Also parents of children and couples worried about fertility issues also want these types of tests. Genetic testing shouldn't be used to screen people out of insurance, employment, or anything else.

Health screening should be focused on matching people to the best possible foods, nutraceuticals, and medicines when and if needed. It should be an inclusive not an exclusive process. Like personnel departments that focus on screening out applicants, genetic testing should not be used to screen people out or to exclude based on genetic risks. Instead, it should be used to draw people into learning about taking responsibility for their own health habits such as choosing the right foods. It's all about choice, like the science of nutrition.

Genetic tests were used on people who suffered from rare genetic disease. Consumers are worried about claims by companies that sell DNA tests to the public. Presently, consumers are asking the FDA to review tests before they are sold to the public or to physicians. The FDA reviews drugs and other medical appliances, why not DNA tests or other health screening tests sold to consumers? Should the government be reviewing these tests?

What do you think? Or should the tests be monitored by the companies offering them? Or should the approach be to the tests similar to vitamins and minerals found in health food stores? What side will you take? Do you have enough information to even begin to take sides? Who runs and regulates the DNA testing companies that may or may not be headed by physicians and geneticists?

Testing DNA for ancestry would not have the same impact on someone's health as testing DNA for a specific disease marker. Still, the people doing the testing should have the same qualifications. What about the people doing the interpreting? What stance do you take? Then there's the question of privacy which is essential.

If you're testing for DNA ancestry, you might want to meet your DNA match to correspond with online. If you're testing for a disease marker, you want privacy. You may want to join a support group of families with similar DNA markers for the specific risk or disease you've inherited. You want meetings held in a hospital or some other private, medical setting. Personal issues come up.

Research the various associations of physicians, such as the American Academy of Family Physicians and other similar groups. You can find opinions there. You can bring in lawyers who want to make sure laws are put into effect to keep employers and insurers from using your results to terminate your job or kick you off of health or life insurance plans if your genes put you at risk.

Set up groups made up of advisories of experts that include consumer groups. What consumers with no science background can do is to work with the US Department of Health and Human Services to monitor various panels of experts. Some people want regulations to change. Others don't. There are hundreds of groups out there who advise the US Dept. of Health on what policies they 'should' adopt.

Consumers ask for reviews. Experts ask for reviews. Consumers don't want their vitamins taken away from health food stores. In the midst of it all are the wonderful DNA tests. Talk to pharmacists as well. If you're having adverse reactions to drugs, you eagerly want a DNA test you can take at home as a consumer.

Genelex Corporation's drug metabolism test can tell you whether your body is taking too long to break down the drugs you're consuming. Consumers need that kind of calmness that comes from knowing personal physicians aren't prescribing too much of what you may or may not need. Maybe you're worrying about your pharmacist giving you the wrong medicine or dosage. Whatever you're concern, a home DNA test is a tool for consumers.

Monitoring your own health is your responsibility, not merely your doctor's. You can get DNA tests sent to your home or scans from clinics. Prescription drugs are available on the Internet. How your body will metabolize what you put into it is important. Are you becoming your own doctor? Is the average consumer becoming more knowledgeable? Or is it more accurate to say most people haven't an inkling of what DNA is?

Pharamcogenetics and nutrigenomics offer tools to consumers. The movement is towards taking charge of your own healthcare. Are doctors worried consumers are taking money away from them? Do tests create more problems than they solve? What happens when scans or other types of tests show non-existent problems?

Research what comes out of the National Institutes of Health. Consumers want to know what the results of their tests mean and how they can apply the information in practical ways. Who interprets the tests? Who is reviewing genetic tests sent directly to consumers and physicians? Right now, it's the consumer's 'job' to ask these questions. If you don't know what vitamins to take, perhaps you need a DNA test to tell you what vitamins work best with your individual genes.

DNA tests seek out mutations in the genes. If a mutation is only remotely associated with a risk, do you ignore it or customize your food and vitamins to the mutation that is only remotely connected to the risk? What action do you take as a consumer? You talk to a physician who knows about genes and your particular risk or you go to a genetics counselor. If you have certain forms of a gene that results in cancer of a certain area of your body by a certain age, you take action right away. Some mutations are associated with disease and some are not, such as certain ancestry markers.

Some genes account for only a tiny percentage of certain cancers. Not everyone needs to be tested. If you have a family reason to be tested, then get tested. If one of your siblings or parents has an inheritable disease, get tested. You can check out Myriad Genetics based in Utah regarding their breast and ovarian cancer tests, available only through doctors. Their Web site is at: http://www.myriad.com/. Or contact them at: Myriad Genetic Laboratories, Inc. | 320 Wakara Way, SLC UT 84108-1214

◆   ◆   ◆

The Controversy and Debate over Whether Genetic Tests should be Sold to the Public

Professionals working in molecular genetics may be divided among those who think genetic tests should be sold to the general consumer and those who think they should not. The professionals who think genetic tests should not be sold to the public may underestimate the intelligence of the public's drive to learn as much as possible about their own genes—the DNA, ancestry, health response to medicine and chemicals in their environment, their response to prescription and over-the-counter drugs, and their response to food, nutraceuticals and other supplements.

Those who are against selling genetic tests to the public fear that genetic testing is way too complex for the average consumer to understand. The average consumer consists of the person who says "it's way over my head," or "my eyes are glazing over" when you mention anything scientific, and the individual who wants to learn as much as possible about his or her own DNA, health, ancestry, and genetic response to food.

Most consumers only need to be told that more than a hundred mutations can cause a specific disorder or disease. Average consumers can understand that. Those who underestimate the intelligence and desire to learn of an individual about his or her own health or the health of children and parents usually are the ones who are first to speak out in censorship of a consumer's right to learn all that is possible to learn at the moment about his own genes.

When a consumer is told that negative results don't always signal health, he or she is intelligent to understand that plain English or any language statement. It's a learning process. Some genetics companies are in direct marketing. Some test DNA only for ancestry. Other genetics companies test for genetic responses to drugs or for various genetic health risks that can be helped by changes in diet. The aim of these companies is cooperation. That means cooperation between patient, physician, genetics counselor, dietician or nutritionist and anyone else involved in the healthcare team working with the patient.

In fact in genetics testing, patients are really clients seeking information, feedback, and recommendations for changes in lifestyle and diet. In drug response genetic testing, the client wants to know how his or her body metabolizes the prescription or over-the-counter medicines used. The whole idea of genetic testing is to bring the healthcare team closer to the healthcare consumer. Instead of a one-size-fits all attitude with drugs, foods, or nutraceuticals, or the usual five to fifteen minute consultation with a doctor, the consumer can have the chance to learn everything publicly available about how his or her genes respond to food, drugs, chemicals in the environment, or lifestyle changes.

If a genetics testing company markets cancer tests, it should have the responsibility to let the patient know that the tests are meant for specific people with specific familial cancers and not for the entire consumer population. When a genetics company takes a family history, it opens doors to the individual not only to explore a familial inherited disease or risk, but the entire history and ancestry of the person's family and the DNA of the family members.

Individuals need to learn that there could be more than one gene involved. So teaching consumers about their DNA and genes is important. Classes could be springing up to train people what to expect before they undergo testing. It's a matter of learning and teaching. This is one more way to make use of retired professionals and other scientists and physicians or genetics counselors working in molecular genetics—helping consumers learn what they can expect from testing.

Consumers need to learn about how important it is to sequence certain genes from many family members. Consumers need to get in touch with affected family members and form a support group for DNA testing, perhaps creating a time capsule for future generations with genetic information resulting from testing.

Most consumers go to their family doctors first. Yet how many family physicians are interested in, let alone trained in molecular genetics? Not so many. Most physicians may not interpret a genetic test correctly because they haven't been trained to do so. In may be that the consumer is the first person to request training be set up to show physicians how to interpret genetic tests, especially for such diseases as cancer. Consumers have more power as a group.

Consumers need to become involved, work together as an organization, and make sure not only the physicians are trained, but also themselves as consumers of genetic testing. Perhaps the physician and consumer can learn together in groups set up for both, where at a point, physician and consumer meet together. Will this present the physician differently in the eyes of the patient? Not really. The science is new enough so that consumer and patient could learn together to unravel the mysteries of genetics not unlike checking the clues in a mystery novel.

Consumers need to read more medical journals such as the New England Journal of Medicine. Spend some time in the library of your local medical school reading about how physicians interpret genetic testing. Look at surveys. As of now, not too many general consumers from the public at large even know what DNA is. So you have to educate yourself, perhaps as a new hobby. First find out what DNA is. Look it up in the dictionary.

Then start reading magazine articles about genetic testing. Look on the Web at the testing companies. Then you can graduate to reading articles in medical journals. The gap between the physician and the consumer needs to be narrowed at least when it comes to your own DNA and genetic testing for the things consumers put into their body such as food and prescribed or over-the-counter medicines, supplements such as herbs, and other nutraceuticals.

Everyone talks about the consumer's consent to testing. The problem is that the consumer needs to be given information. If you're going to eat 'smarter' you have to become informed first. If you have an inheritable risk or disease, you need to understand everything you can find that is publicly accessible about the risk, the disease, or the genes involved.

Material is online, but is it credible? There are always the articles in medical journals, but can you understand the terminology? If not, look up the terms in glossaries and dictionaries. Make a list of terms and learn how to make the journal articles understandable in plain language.

Think about risk for a moment. Your risk could change. How are you going to receive the information from genetic testing? What are you going to do about it as far as changing your lifestyle, diet, or medicines?

If you are concerned how your family might react to genetic testing, ask them whether they would change their food choices or other lifestyle changes based on the information. You can always keep the information private, but it could save the lives of family members to get tested and to change what can be changed, such as food choices or exercise routines.

Most consumers worry more about discrimination in employment and health insurance due to companies finding out their genetic risks. Privacy must be kept, and information only given to the consumer of the testing, not his employer or health insurance company. It's nobody's business but your own as far as your genetic information. So, measures to keep out strangers from using your genes against you must be in order. That's why numbers instead of names work better with testing.

The big issue is accuracy. If so many physicians cannot correctly interpret a genetic test and advise their patients, more training is needed for the physicians and the patients. It's a case of whose watching the watchers.

Who is going to review the genetic testing itself as to accuracy? What if the tests are not accurate? Right now nobody is reviewing the testing companies other than themselves. Nobody is reporting directly to the consumer after checking the accuracy of the genetic tests. And nobody is reporting directly to the physician with that same information.

If you're going to get tested, at least learn as much as most professional genetic counselors know about interpreting your tests. It can be done without going back to school for a graduate degree in molecular genetics.

The information is available to the public from libraries, the Internet, databases, and medical school libraries, journals, and professional articles. Many are on the Web in PDF files. Subscribe to the journals or read them in libraries and learn how to interpret your own tests. Then form a consumer's group to watch the watchers. Learn how to check the accuracy of tests done by the testing companies.

You have to become involved in your own healthcare and nutrition. Take charge and take responsibility. Consumers can't be passive. You won't know how your body responds to food or medicine or lifestyle changes until symptoms appear. Start by looking at the health of your family members and realizing what is inheritable, and what you can do to help yourself if you've inherited what they have or will get.

The first step for consumers is to start learning about DNA and genetic testing just as they have learned about genealogy and family history. Classes online or in adult education can be set up as well as support groups and organizations of consumers. The second step is to form a group to review the accuracy of information that comes with your genetic tests. Invite physicians and other healthcare professionals to join with consumers and become a team. Don't let separation between those with scientific knowledge and those without become a barrier to reviewing accuracy of information.

When physicians or geneticists band together to review the accuracy of information provided with genetic testing, what might happen is that the group then becomes made up only of professionals. When consumers group together, they can include professionals, but would never ban someone from the group because of professional training in the field they are watching.

So consumers need to create a group to review the accuracy of information that comes with genetic tests. And that same group needs to make sure education exists for consumers. You need to set up classes to train consumers in how to understand the results of their genetic testing and how to review the accuracy of the information given along with the genetic tests.

If trained physicians can't correctly interpret a genetic test for their patients in certain cases, it's time for consumers to take charge of their own healthcare education. Okay, you can't do surgery on yourself, but you can learn to read the information provided with genetic tests. And having read the information, you can learn also to question the accuracy of that information.

Consumers can read not only the medical journal articles usually found in medical school and university libraries open to the public, publications such as the ***New England Journal of Medicine***, but also some of the more popular articles in magazines that go to physicians such as ***Physician's Weekly***. All this autodidact education can be achieved with consumers involvement and support groups if people are interested enough to involve a wide range of members or participants.

Genetic information, research findings, and training at various levels for the press, students, and public should be available to everyone equally. Reliable, scientifically substantiated information needs to be widely available through the Internet, through senior centers, classrooms focused on adult education, through hospitals, libraries, and HMO programs, and through the genetic testing companies.

Doctors' Point/Counterpoint

In the magazine, *Physician's Weekly*, October 7, 2002, Vol. XIX, No. 38, the article in Point/Counterpoint, titled, *"Should genetic tests be sold directly to the public?"* featured Howard Coleman, CEO, Genelex Corp., Redmond, Washington and Kimberly A. Quaid, PhD, Professor of Clinical, Medical, and Molecular Genetics, Clinical Psychiatry, and Clinical Medicine, Indiana University School of Medicine. Coleman's response was yes, and Quaid's response was no. See the article, copyrighted 2002 by *Physician's Weekly*, reprinted below with permission.

Should genetic tests be sold directly to the public?

Howard Coleman, CEO, Genelex Corp., Redmond, Washington.

YES Every person has the right to know his or her genetic information, and the right not to share it. People have legitimate privacy concerns about their genetic information being loose in the medical records system, fearing for their jobs or insurance if it gets into the wrong hands. Physicians are also concerned, and don't want to risk compromising a patient's privacy. This contributes to their reluctance to order genetic tests.

There are compelling reasons for people to obtain reliable genetic information, whether they go through their doctors or not. According to a 1998 JAMA article, more than 100,000 deaths occur annually due to adverse drug reactions, along with an additional 2.2 million serious events that require hospital stays. These are not medical mishaps, as they occur within the labeled use of drugs.

When physicians begin to learn the genotype of their patients they will begin to solve this problem. The practice of their clinical art will be improved because in many instances the genotype of their patient trumps the many other characteristics they do know.

Despite the facts that science has known for the past half century that people react differently to drugs, doctors have been unable to put genetic testing into practice for the benefit of their patients. Doctors lack sufficient training in pharmacogenetics and drug metabolism. For example, most doctors don't know that genotyping for Coumadin metabolism is available, and that it will help patients avoid adverse reactions with this drug.

Adverse drug reactions kill many people in the U.S., but the threat goes largely unrecognized. Making gene tests available directly to patients not only provides a valuable service, but helps push the medical community into the 21st century era of personalized and evidence-based medicine.

Kimberly A. Quaid, PhD, Professor of Clinical, Medical, and Molecular Genetics, Clinical Psychiatry, and Clinical Medicine Indiana University School of Medicine

NO No. Genetic testing is far too complex for lay people to tackle on their own. For example, more than 100 mutations can cause cystic fibrosis, and most genetic tests only cover a small subset of these. But most lay people don't understand that negative results are not necessarily a clean bill of health.

The announcement last spring that Myriad Genetics would direct market cancer tests was particularly troubling, because such tests are only appropriate for a small number of individuals with certain familial cancers. The complex protocol includes taking a detailed family history, then finding and sequencing the gene from affected relatives (and there may be more than one gene).

Individuals who hear about such tests might approach their family physicians, but research shows that many are not trained in genetics. A paper in the NEJM, which looked at physicians ordering a test for a particular cancer, found that one third of these physicians interpreted the test incorrectly. One can assume that if physicians have trouble interpreting the results, patients will fare far worse. One survey found that fewer than 26% of Americans know what DNA is.

Geneticists believe testing should be preceded by informed consent. For consent to be informed, the patient must understand the disorder for which they are being tested, their current risk, how their risk might change as a result of testing, the ramifications of their being tested for their families and spouses, and the possibility of discrimination should third parties get their hands on this information.

Finally, no mechanism exists to review the accuracy of information provided with genetic tests to either health-care professionals or consumers. Individuals who get tested without professional counseling may buy trouble with their test results.

In our recent email interview of August 19, 2003, Howard Coleman added, "I agree with Dr. Quaid when the testing concerns the grave medical conditions caused by genetic disease and we don't offer those tests to the general public. The testing we do provide can help both the physician and the individual understand their ability to metabolize drugs which can help to prevent adverse drug reactions and how to optimize their diet."

Scientists and Physicians Comment on Pharmacogenetics

Why would the average consumer of health care want to have drug reaction testing, known as pharmacogenetic testing? The field is new, and still emerging. According to (reprinted with permission) Genelex's "Health and DNA" Web site (copyright 2003) at: http://www.healthanddna.com/, "The relatively new and emerging fields of pharmacogenetics studies how differences in individual genetic makeup affect the processing of drugs. We have known for about a half-century that individuals respond to the same drug and dosage in very different ways because of genetic variations called polymorphisms. Research shows that of all the clinical factors such as age, sex, weight, general health and liver function that alter a patient's response to drugs, genetic factors are the most important.

Genelex is the first firm in the world to offer genetic drug reaction testing directly to the public." Genelex also offers DNA testing for **nutritional** genetics, drug reaction testing, ancestry-based DNA testing, and DNA identity testing.

DNA traditionally had been used to identify people, mostly in forensic or paternity or relationship cases. Then a few years ago, companies began to test DNA for ancestry, which appeals also to genealogists, family historians, and oral historians. The use of DNA outside of court rooms and forensic laboratories and outside of government and university databases brought DNA to consumers of health care as well as to genealogists interested in molecular genealogy.

University laboratories and archaeology research institutes began using the science of archaeogenetics. Anthropologists who looked at HLA markers, those leukocytes or white blood cells and physicians or scientists who were interested in tissue typing for blood, marrow, and organ transplant donors worked with DNA to identify similar matches, people whose tissues and blood or marrow typing matched close enough for a transplant to take.

You had scientists who studied ancient DNA from fossils and mummies expand the science of archaeogenetics and population geneticists studying migrations of ancient peoples and the routes they took. When ancient and present day comparisons of genetic markers left trails that matched with archaeological relics, new branches of molecular genetics grew.

The science is still emerging, using DNA testing in more ways. Now, we have nutrition and genetics and drug testing and genetics. And there's so much more to arrive that will be available to the general consumer of healthcare, ancestry searching, and identity. From being a spectator in life watching new avenues of

DNA testing unfold, the consumer now has the chance to become more involved in participating in and learning about how many ways DNA testing can benefit an individual at any age.

Go to Genelex's Web site to explore more material on DNA testing for a variety of purposes. The consumer has more choices than ever before and still more on the horizon. Is DNA testing all about nourishment?

From nutrigenomics to drug reaction testing, strategies for better health are being covered from all angles. Perhaps you—as a consumer—want a healthier eating guideline customized to your genetic signature.

Maybe you'd like a report on how your genes (and body) respond to certain chemicals, medicines, or substances. Whether it's a prescription drug or specific medicines or supplements that you buy over the counter, several genes are tested to see how your body metabolizes the substance. Not every gene in your body is tested to see how they respond to food or medicine—just specific genes and markers.

The science is new and changing, but the future is attractive to general consumers. You don't need a science background to begin your research on how your own body responds to what you put into it and what comes it from the environment.

To begin, consumers need to become more involved in learning about what scientists and physicians are researching and why, and how all these new findings apply to you. To become more involved as a consumer means being able to access information that evaluates the research, that finds credibility or flaws, and that helps you take more responsibility in your own maintenance.

Can genetic testing can open doors in the fields of nutrition and pharmacogenetics? Even with guarded caution, the benefits are to be explored and discussed.

If you have already had your DNA tested for ancestry or identity, consider these new ways in which DNA testing can help you draw up a plan for eating and for any way you take care of your body—from exercise planning and nutrition to medicines and supplements if and when you need them, to making lifestyle changes for better health.

Consumers can learn a lot from news releases, including learning to understand where to begin to educate themselves about their genes. Some of these releases come from universities engaged in research, some from laboratories and genetic testing companies, some from the government, and from other scientific sources.

Professionals in molecular genetics and in healthcare need to understand that an open door policy for public education, teaching oneself about DNA is good.

To become more informed leads to becoming more involved in consumer's groups for understanding what "gene hunters" are doing.

Science has become so technical that most scientific journal articles are not understood by most consumers without science training. There has to be a mid-way point. So far, it's the media that translates scientific terminology into plain language for the consumer. Going one step farther, the medical journalist translates the scientific journals into articles and books whereby people with no science background can learn about their genes.

Finally, learning about how one's genes respond to food or drugs is another rung up on the ladder of self-education about how your body works. That's why there's the mass media for the consumer, the popular medical magazines that bring the consumer closer to healthcare professionals, and finally, the scientific and medical journal articles discussing the research. At the top are the evaluators who let the consumers know which research studies were flawed, and that usually filters down through the mass media.

What some scientists call 'snake oil' may either be harmful or may be a forgotten remedy based on plants that worked. For example, honey, cinnamon, and sesame oil. All three will resist bacteria and in the ancient past were used on minor wounds. A century ago colloidal silver was used on scratches to keep out bacteria.

In the Civil War days, it was used on wounds. Today, you can still make your own, inexpensively, but be careful buying brands containing aluminum. In the dentist's chair, colloidal silver mouthwash works as well as some of the more recent remedies such as washing your mouth with harsh substances that can cause ulcers in the mouth.

The point is to check out the mechanisms that review accuracy in whatever you read. If you go the homeopathic or naturopathic route, make sure what you use does no harm for your individual genetic response. How do you metabolize what goes into your body? Genetic testing can help here.

When it comes to genetic testing, can you learn a lot from news releases—at least as a starting point in your research and education about your genes? Bio-science communicators have a role to play as interpreters between consumer and scientist. In genetics, being the communicator means bridging the gap between the growing body of knowledge in science and the consumer who might not even know what DNA is.

If you have no science knowledge, start by using press releases as a way to formulate questions to ask librarians in order to find more information. Open the first set of doors to understand more about how nutrition is related to your genetic markers, and DNA. What can news releases disseminated by corporations tell you about science?

◆   ◆   ◆

What Consumers Can Learn From News Releases
NIGMS Awards $35 Million To UCSD-Led Consortium To Map Metabolic Pathways In Cells

According to a UCSD media release of August 11, 2003, the University of California, San Diego (UCSD) will lead an ambitious national effort to produce a detailed understanding of the structure and function of lipids—cellular fats and oils implicated in a wide range of diseases, including heart disease, stroke, cancer, diabetes and Alzheimer's disease.

The five-year, $35 million grant from the National Institute of General Medical Sciences (NIGMS) will support more than 30 researchers at 18 universities, medical research institutes, and companies across the United States, who will work together in a detailed analysis of the structure and function of lipids. The principal investigator of this collaboration is Edward Dennis, Ph.D, professor of chemistry and biochemistry in UCSD's Division of Physical Sciences and UCSD's School of Medicine.

Dennis notes that while sequencing the human genome was a scientific landmark, it is just the first step in understanding the diverse array of systems and processes within and among cells. Establishment of this consortium is a significant step in an emerging field called "metabolomics," or the study of metabolites, chemical compounds that "turn on or off cellular responses to food, friend, or foe," he explained.

Lipids are a water-insoluble subset of metabolites central to the regulation and control of normal cellular function, and to disease. Stored as an energy reserve for the cell, lipids are vital components of the cell membrane, and are involved in communication within and between cells. For example, one class of lipids, the sterols, includes estrogen and testosterone.

The initial phases of the project, known as Lipid Metabolites And Pathways Strategy (LIPID MAPS), will be aimed at characterizing all of the lipid metabolites in one type of cell. The term "Lipidomics" is used to describe the study of lipids and their complex changes and interactions within cells. Because this task is too extensive for a single laboratory to complete, researchers at participating centers will each focus on isolating and characterizing all of the lipids in a single class.

This information will then be combined into a database at <http://www. lipidmaps.org> to identify networks of interactions amongst lipid metabolites and to make this information available to other researchers. Shankar Subramaniam, Ph.D., professor of chemistry and bioengineering at UCSD's Jacobs School of Engineering and San Diego Supercomputer Center, will coordinate this aspect of the project.

The cell type selected for study is the macrophage, best known for its role in immune reactions, for example scavenging bacteria and other invaders in the body. Macrophage cells from mice will be used, rather than human cells, because there exists a "library" of mouse cells with specific genetic mutations.

By studying cells missing certain genes, the research team will attempt to identify what genes code for those enzymes key in synthesis and processing of lipid metabolites. Christopher Glass, M.D., Ph.D., professor of cellular and molecular medicine at UCSD's School of Medicine, will coordinate the macrophage biology and genomics aspects of the consortium.

According to Dennis, one of the most difficult aspects of this project will be to ensure that all the participating research sites are using identical methods. "There has never been an effort to detect all the lipid metabolites in a cell and to quantify the amounts of these lipids," says Dennis. "In order to be able take the data gathered by each lab and put them together to develop new ideas about interactions between lipid metabolites, it is essential to develop new technologies and methods and to standardize them so that they can be applied in the same way at each research site."

Once the researchers have developed these methods and used them to identify and quantify the lipid metabolites in the mouse macrophage, the methods can be applied to gather other information about lipid metabolites in cells. The researchers plan to study the time and dose-dependent effects of lipopolysaccharide, or LPS, a component of the cell walls of many bacteria, on macrophages.

Dennis' lab has studied the effects of LPS on macrophages for the last 20 years. A world authority on these effects, Dennis says that this large-scale, cross-institutional collaboration will create an understanding of LPS' effects on lipid metabolism in unprecedented detail, and set the stage for examining other macrophage effectors such as oxidized LDL, the so-called bad cholesterol which leads to atherosclerosis.

A detailed understanding of lipid metabolism will be valuable in drug design. Most people are already familiar with one class of drugs that interfere with lipid metabolism: the non-steroidal anti-inflammatory drugs (NSAIDs), which include aspirin and ibuprofen. These drugs block the synthesis of prostaglandins, a large group of chemicals secreted by macrophages that causes pain, inflammation and an immunological response.

Statins, which a large number of Americans take daily to lower their cholesterol levels, also dramatically alter lipid metabolites. With a detailed knowledge of each step in the lipid metabolic pathways, more effective drugs with fewer side effects can be designed to combat heart disease and a plethora of other diseases of lipid metabolism.

In addition to UCSD, participants in the LIPID MAPS consortium are: Avanti Polar Lipids, Inc.; Duke University Medical School; Georgia Institute of Technology; University of California, Irvine; University of Colorado School of Medicine; University of Texas Southwestern Medical School; and Vanderbilt University Medical School. Additional collaborators will include scientists from Applied Biosystems; Boston University School of Medicine; Harvard Medical School; Medical College of Georgia; Medical University of South Carolina; National Jewish Medical and Research Center; Scripps Research Institute; University of Michigan Medical School; University of Utah; and Virginia Commonwealth University. For more information on the grant program, see the related release at http://www.nigms.nih.gov/news/releases/.

DNA testing isn't only for geneticists and anthropologists. It includes but goes beyond forensic research in identity. It expands from population genetics to cellular nourishment. It's for the general consumer with no science training, the physician, the genetics counselor, and the nutritionist. DNA testing is for the genealogist and the oral historian. And there are many more applications of DNA testing/genetic testing on the horizon.

Genelex and How Your Body Processes Medicines

According to Genelex's Web site (copyright 2003) at: http://www. healthanddna.com/pharmacogenetics.html, (reprinted below with permission):

The relatively new and emerging fields of pharmacogenetics and pharmacogenomics study how differences in individual genetic makeup affect the processing of drugs. Pharmacogenetics largely focuses on specific genes, such as drug-metabolizing enzymes, while pharmacogenomics deals with the entire human genome, including genes for numerous proteins in the body, such as transporters, receptors, and the entire signaling networks that respond to drugs and move them through the system.

We have known for about a half-century that individuals respond to the same drug and dosage in very different ways because of genetic variations called polymorphisms. The first studies of what came to be pharmacogenetics were conducted in the early 1950s and examined drug metabolizing enzyme variants such as those in the Cytochrome P450 family. Research shows that of all the clinical factors such as age, sex, weight, general health and liver function that alter a patient's response to drugs, genetic factors are the most important.

Although the genomes of individuals are 99.9% identical, the 0.1% difference means we have as many as 3 million polymorphisms, the most common being the single nucleotide polymorphism (SNP). Detecting polymorphisms is the foundation of pharmacogenetics.

Misdosing of drugs in America costs more than $100 billion dollars a year, and is a leading cause of death. Pharmacogenetics helps to explain why some individuals respond to drugs and others don't. It can also help doctors identify individuals needing higher or lower doses and who will respond to a drug therapeutically and who might have an adverse drug reaction.

Currently, the clinical use of pharmacogenetics is limited, with the most extensive use in Scandinavia to treat psychiatric illnesses. The technology is, however, steadily moving into other geographic and medical areas, especially cardiology and cancer treatment.

The Human Genome Project has been an incredible boon to pharmacogenomics. As new data are decoded and more precise maps produced, we can begin to understand what specific genes are and how they function. We can also better appreciate the significance of DNA variation among individuals. Preventative medicine and pharmacogentics are the first disciplines to benefit from this vastly increased understanding of human diversity.

Better understanding of the variation in the enzymes involved in drug metabolism and in the drug targets themselves will help explain why there is so much variation in drug response. We are now able to test for these variations before prescribing, and reduce the amount of human experimentation (and associated health care costs) needed to find the best therapy or dose. Drug companies can now develop drugs which are designed by choice, rather than happenstance, to be effective in wide range of the population.

Predictive genetics is revolutionizing health care. DNA tests and personalized drug therapies are shifting the medical paradigm from detection and treatment to prediction and prevention and vastly increasing the efficacy, safety, and variety of therapeutic drugs. Predictive tests and preventative therapies reduce costs associated with hospitalization and lost productivity and will lead to a major redistribution of value in the health care industry."

Also, according to the **Genelex** Web site at: http://www.healthanddna.com/drugreactiontest.html, (reprinted below with permission, copyright Genelex 2003.)

Drug Reaction Testing

Do not alter the dosage amount or schedule of any drug you are taking without first consulting your doctor or pharmacist. Research shows that of all the clinical factors such as age, sex, weight, general health and liver function that alter a patient's response to drugs, genetic factors are the most important. This information becomes even more crucial when you consider the fact that adverse reactions to prescription drugs are killing about 106,000 Americans each year—roughly three times as many as are killed by automobiles. This makes prescription drugs the fourth leading killer in the U.S., after heart disease, cancer, and stroke."

We currently offer CYP2D6, CYP2C9, and CYP2C19 screens that can help your physician or druggist predict your particular response to more than a quarter of all prescription drugs. These include such important medications as Coumadin (Warfarin), Prozac, Zoloft, Paxil, Effexor, Hydrocodone, Amitriptyline, Claritin, Cyclobenzaprine, Haldol, Metoprolol, Rythmol, Tagamet, Tamoxifen, Valium, Carisoprodol, Diazepam, Dilantin, Premarin, and Prevacid (and the over-the-counter drugs, Allegra, Dytuss and Tusstat). Click here to view a more complete list of drugs processed through these pathways."

Approximately half of all Americans have genetic defects that affect how they process these drugs. There are four different types of metabolizers, and we all fall into one of these categories for the variable pathways in Cytochrome P450 (this Cytochrome is responsible for creating the enzymes that process chemicals of all kinds through our bodies.) The easiest way to understand this is to picture a two lane highway.

If you are the first type which is the norm, you would be an EXTENSIVE metabolizer. Both lanes of the highway are open and moving. Medications prescribed in normal doses will be metabolized by your body.

If you are the second type, you would be an INTERMEDIATE metabolizer. This means that one lane of that highway is open and moving and the other lane is not, causing you to metabolize the medications more slowly. In this case you will need a lower dosage, and there is a chance of medications building up in your system causing adverse effects. It is especially important to monitor medications if you are in this category.

Intermediate metabolizers through the 2C9 pathway, for instance, have an increased risk of bleeding incidences when taking the common blood thinner

Coumadin or Warfarin. For this reason, a recent article in the Journal of the American Medical Association, titled "*Association Between CYP2C9 Genetic Variants and Anticoagulation-Related Outcomes During Wayfarin Therapy*," JAMA, April 3, 2002—Vol. 287, No. 13, recommends screening for CYP2C9 variants to reduce the risk of adverse drug reactions in these patients.

The third type is a POOR metabolizer. In this case both lanes of the highway would be stopped. There is a possiblility that alternate routes can be found, but this type of metabolizer is potentially very dangerous, as there is a great chance for the medication to build up in your system making you very sick, or even killing you. For example, a poor metabolizer of Phenytoin, a common antiepileptic would not be able to process the drug and would actually have an increased rather than decreased risk of seizure if prescribed this drug.

The fourth type of metabolizer is ULTRA EXTENSIVE. This means you have additional lanes for processing, picture an Indy 500 speedway. In this instance, you literally burn through medications. If you were an Ultra extensive metabolizer through the 2D6 pathway and while in surgery and your doctor gave you codeine as a pain killer, you would receive no pain relief because the codeine would be metabolized so fast that it would have little or no effect on you.

The Testing Process

The process is simple. We send you a blood collection kit in the mail. You can either make an appointment with your doctor or we will provide you with the contact information for a phlebotomist in your area. Blood samples are overnighted to our laboratory and results are typically available in 15 business days.

Currently Available Tests

CYP2D6 (cytochrome P450 2D6) is the best studied of the DMEs and acts on one-fourth of all prescription drugs, including the selective serotonin reuptake inhibitors (SSRI), tricylic antidepressants (TCA), betablockers such as Inderal and the Type 1A antiarrhythmics. Approximately 10% of the population has a slow acting form of this enzyme and 7% a super-fast acting form. Thirty-five percent are carriers of a non-functional 2D6 allele, especially elevating the risk of ADRs when these individuals are taking multiple drugs.

Drugs that CYP2D6 metabolizes include Prozac, Zoloft, Paxil, Effexor, Hydrocodone, Amitriptyline, Claritin, Cyclobenzaprine, Haldol, Metoprolol, Rythmol, Tagamet, Tamoxifen, and the over-the-counter diphenylhydramine drugs, Allegra, Dytuss, and Tusstat. CYP2D6 is responsible for activating the pro-drug codeine into its active form and the drug is therefore inactive in CYP2D6 slow metabolizers.

CYP2C9 (cytochrome P450 2C9) is the primary route of metabolism for Coumadin (Warfarin). Approximately 10% of the population are carriers of at least one allele for the slow-metabolizing form of CYP2C9 and may be treatable with 50% of the dose at which normal metabolizers are treated. Other drugs metabolized by CYP2C9 include Amaryl, Isoniazid, Sulfa, Ibuprofen, Amitriptyline, Dilantin, Hyzaar, THC (tetrahydrocannabinol), Naproxen, and Viagra.

CYP2C19 (cytochrome P450 2C19) is associated with the metabolism of Carisoprodol, Diazepam, Dilantin, Premarin, and Prevacid.

Other tests in the planning stage at the time this book went to press include: **NAT2** (N-acetyltransferase 2) is a second-step DME that acts on Isoniazid, Procainamide, and Azulfidine. The frequency of the NAT2 "slow acetylator" in various worldwide populations ranges from 10% to more than 90%.

The advantages of Genelex's consumer genetic testing include:

Safety. Decrease the chance that you will be the victim of an adverse drug reaction. More than 100,000 hospitalized Americans die of adverse drug reactions and two million outpatients have serious episodes each year. Knowledge of your DNA Drug Reaction Profile may help your physician or druggist prevent this from happening.

Efficacy. Prescription drugs on the market today are usually prescribed by trial and error because they have been tested and approved in a "one size fits all" fashion. If you eliminate a particular drug more rapidly than the norm, taking the normal dose may be a complete waste of time. The drug simply will not work as prescribed, and it may take a while to discover this.

Responsibility. Play a more active role in your health, your family's health, and in healthcare at large. DNA testing for drug reactions is just coming onto the market and you, the consumer, can help all of us take this major step toward better medicine."

Check out the common drugs processed by enzymes that Genelex tests. Genelex currently offers "DNA Prescription Drug Reaction Profiles" that test 2D6,2C9, and 2c19 functionality. Look at Genelex's many commonly prescribed drugs such as those listed at their Web site or in their literature that are metabolized through these pathways in the Cytochrome P-450 system. If your medication is not on the list, ask your pharmacist or physician to explain to you the facts you should know as a consumer about the metabolic pathway.

Food and Medicines Are Processed by Enzymes

Common drugs prescribed by physicians or bought over-the-counter are processed by enzymes. Look at Genelex's Drug List by clicking on the PDF file to see Genelex's Drug list. Go to their Web site at: http://www.healthanddna.com/ drugreactiontest.html and click on the PDF file to view the list of drugs at: http://www.healthanddna.com/drugchart.PDF.

What you're looking for is prescription drug reaction testing. Your body metabolizes drugs differently than another person based on your individual genetic response. So look at the drug metabolization guide. Is your prescription drug listed there? What about drugs or supplements you buy over the counter? The typeset formatting is different on the PDF file. So look at the list below at: http://www.healthanddna.com/drugchart.PDF.

On the PDF file, you'll note that the formatting for numbers such as 2D6 is different in the PDF file than reprinted here due to formatting differences between a paperback book and the PDF file on the Web.

So to get the correct formatting of the numbers such as 2D6 lined up with the correct drugs, use the PDF file to do your looking rather than the book, which is just a list of drugs tested. The PDF file has the correct numbers lined up with the correct names of the drugs.

Find out what drug reaction testing is about and the names of the drugs listed. Look at Genelex's PDF file if you want to see what numbers are lined up with what drugs. Ask your physician or pharmacist or a pharmacogeneticist how a drug metabolization guide may be of benefit to a consumer when talking to your physician.

The point is for you to learn how to become more involved in researching how your genes respond to what you put in your body, be it food, skin care products, or medicine. Personalized medicine and predictive medicine may involve genetic, metabolic, and body-type testing, nutrition, and customizing diets and activities according to your genetic signature. Each professional may specialize in a particular area of personalized medicine.

◆   ◆   ◆

Debating Vitamin E Controversies

How do you write a scientific article or outline a debate intended for the mass media, consumers, students and educators? When organizing your debate or term paper on the issues surrounding vitamin E and its effects, check out the articles online posted by the International Food Information Council.

These informative articles offer discussions in plain language. For example, one excellent issue in the media to debate concerns the health effects of vitamin E. When you read the article reprinted below, note how easy to read the article is because it is written in plain language.

The article below still contains the scientific study results presented in a way that is easily understandable by students, consumers, and health-care professionals. Communication shares meaning. The article on the health effects of vitamin E is reprinted here with the permission of the International Food Information Council. This article also appears online at: http://ific.org/foodinsight/2005/ja/vitaminefi405.cfm

◆   ◆   ◆

The Health Effects of Vitamin E: A Case Study in Communicating Emerging Science

---

Food Insight
July/August 2005

A recent study in the *Journal of the American Medical Association* (*JAMA*) looked at major studies cited by scientists over a 13-year period and found that, because of the developing nature of science and research, 16 percent of the time these studies were contradicted by subsequent research findings. The *JAMA* study underscores the fact that science is, and should be, evolutionary in order to enhance our understanding of an issue.

One of the latest debates in nutrition research involves the use of vitamin E possibly to reduce the risk of or delay chronic disease. Evidence has suggested that this potent antioxidant may lower the risk for various diseases, including heart disease, some types of cancer, cataracts, age-related macular degeneration, Parkinson's disease, and Alzheimer's disease.

Yet, some recent research has cast doubt on the safety and efficacy of vitamin E dietary supplements—once heralded as a "golden child" of antioxidants—causing debate among scientists as to the merits of supplemental vitamin E.

Antioxidant Abilities

The theory behind the role of antioxidants in good health is well known. Certain nutrients are believed to slow or prevent oxidative damage in the body, which is implicated in the development of many diseases. Dr. Jeffrey Blumberg, a professor in the Friedman School of Nutrition Science and Policy and Director of the Antioxidants Research Laboratory at Jean Mayer USDA Human Nutrition Research Center on Aging, believes that the antioxidant theory related to disease prevention is strong, yet not definitive. "There is provocative evidence from animal studies and observational studies with humans that antioxidants such as vitamin E may be helpful in preventing disease," says Blumberg. "But current research does not support the use of antioxidants in a therapeutic role."

Herein lies the challenge with communicating the results of vitamin E research. According to Dr. Takayuki Shibamoto, a professor in the Department of Environmental Toxicology at the University of California, Davis, one reason that recent studies with vitamin E have produced discouraging results is because some overestimate the power of vitamin E. "Antioxidants do not have drug-like abilities," says Shibamoto. Rather, he explains that antioxidants are better suited to help reduce the risk or slow the progression of disease so other body processes or medications can better fight the disease.

Vitamin E is a case in point—illustrating that with any research, new evidence needs to be considered carefully before making generalized recommendations or discounting the results of previous well-conducted research. This article will help to put today's knowledge of vitamin E into context.

Background on Vitamin E

This fat-soluble vitamin found in plants exists in eight different forms. The forms vary in their biological activity, or potency, in the body. In its natural form of alpha-tocopherol, vitamin E is most biologically active in humans and also functions as an antioxidant.

Many vitamin E supplements are synthetic and derived from petroleum, while the natural form comes mainly from soybean oil. On a dietary supplement label, the simplest way to determine which form is used is to look at the ingredients: "dl"-alpha-tocopherol means synthetic; "d" instead of "dl" means it's natural.

The Institute of Medicine (IOM) established a Recommended Dietary Allowance (RDA) for vitamin E as part of the Dietary Reference Intakes (see Table 1). The RDA for vitamin E is provided as "alpha-tocopherol equivalents" or ATEs, to account for the different biological activities of the varying forms of vitamin E. Foods and some supplements that label vitamin E will list the amount in International Units (IU) because the Daily Value for vitamin E is measured in IUs. The Daily Value for vitamin E is 30 IUs (or 20 mg ATE).

The IOM set a Tolerable Upper Intake Level (UL) for vitamin E at 1000 mg per day (1,500 IU natural vitamin E; 1,000 IU synthetic vitamin E) of supplementary alpha-tocopherol for adults. The UL is the highest daily intake likely to pose no risk of adverse health effects to almost all individuals in the general population. Due to its anticoagulant properties, bleeding problems were the adverse health effect or "critical endpoint" on which to base the UL for vitamin E.

Common food sources of vitamin E include vegetable oils, nuts, green leafy vegetables, and fortified cereals. National surveys suggest that the diets of most Americans do not meet the recommended intake for vitamin E. The Dietary Guidelines for Americans identify vitamin E as a nutrient for concern because intake levels are believed to be low in adults and children.

Evidence for Vitamin E

Related to heart disease, vitamin E is believed to inhibit oxidative changes to LDL ("bad") cholesterol that promote blockages in blood vessels leading to heart attack and stroke. Observational and clinical studies support this hypothesis.

An observational study of approximately 90,000 nurses suggested that incidence of heart disease was 30% to 40% lower among nurses with the highest intake of vitamin E from diet and supplements. The apparent benefit was mainly derived from vitamin E supplements because high intake of vitamin E from food alone was not associated with cardiac risk reduction. Similarly, a 1993 study of 40,000 male health professionals found those who took at least 100 IUs daily for two years had a third fewer cases of heart disease than those receiving no vitamin E supplements. A 1996 study from the National Institutes on Aging followed 11,000 elderly people for seven years and found the death rate for vitamin E users was a third of that of nonusers.

In an intervention study, the Cambridge Heart Antioxidant Study (CHAOS), researchers assigned 2,002 participants with established heart disease to receive either 800 IU or 400 IU of vitamin E or a placebo for a median of 510 days. Treatment with vitamin E substantially reduced the rate of non-fatal heart attack, with beneficial effects apparent after one year. Over a three-year period of vitamin E and vitamin C supplementation in men and postmenopausal women 45-69 years with elevated blood cholesterol levels, researchers in Finland observed a 74% reduction of atherosclerotic progression in men.

Vitamin E may also play a role in cancer risk reduction by protecting against free radicals implicated in cancer, blocking the formation of cancer-promoting nitrosamines, and helping to enhance immune function. Although research is limited, some studies associate higher intakes of vitamin E with a decreased incidence of specific types of cancer, such as prostate, breast, bladder, and colon. Evidence for a link between vitamin E and prostate cancer was compelling enough to be investigated in a large ongoing clinical trial of 35,000 men.

The National Institutes of Health launched the SELECT study (Selenium and Vitamin E Cancer Prevention Trial) to examine whether one or both of these dietary supplements may help reduce risk of prostate cancer. Other studies are underway to examine the potential benefits of vitamin E in reducing the risk of developing cataracts, age-related macular degeneration, Parkinson's disease, and Alzheimer's disease.

For example, the National Eye Institute launched a new study following the release of promising findings from the Age-Related Eye Disease Study (AREDS), a study of nearly 5,000 participants that found slower progression of age-related macular degeneration with a daily dose of vitamin E (400 IU), beta-carotene, vitamin C, zinc, and copper. The new study will examine if vitamin E, together with lutein and omega-3 fats, can slow the onset of age-related macular degeneration.

Questions Raised about Vitamin E

Recent data from the Women's Health Study, in which nearly 20,000 healthy, middle-aged women were given 600 international units of vitamin E every other day for roughly 10 years, suggest that vitamin E provides no overall benefit for major cardiovascular-related events or cancer, nor does it affect total mortality or decrease cardiovascular-related deaths in healthy women. However, this double-blind, placebo-controlled trial also found that although overall there was no statistically significant cardiovascular benefit to vitamin E, there was a 24 percent reduction in cardiovascular deaths and a 26 percent reduction in major cardiovascular events among a sub-group of women who were 65 or older.

Another randomized clinical trial known as the Heart Outcomes Prevention Evaluation (HOPE) Study found a lack of protection with vitamin E supplements. This study followed nearly 10,000 patients 55 years and older with vascular disease or diabetes. After about five years, the study was extended and renamed HOPE-TOO (HOPE—The Ongoing Outcomes) with nearly 7,000 patients for four more years. The subjects who received 400 IU of vitamin E daily did not experience fewer major cardiovascular events or differences in cancer incidence, but were 13 percent more likely to develop heart failure compared to those not taking vitamin E. Researchers speculated that higher doses of vitamin E may disturb the balance of beneficial, naturally occurring antioxidants.

A review of 19 clinical trials conducted between 1993 and 2004 also found a lack of benefit associated with vitamin E supplements, especially at higher doses. With vitamin E supplements above 400 IU per day, researchers concluded that there was an increased risk for death among older, high-risk patients. This review may be somewhat limited in that it excluded studies reporting fewer than 10 deaths and did not consider the results of epidemiologic observational studies.

Not the Final Word on Vitamin E

Experts suggest there is good reason to be cautious about generalizing the findings of recent vitamin E studies. Blumberg points out that many studies with negative results were secondary prevention trials where study participants were older with existing disease. "The evidence simply does not support the use of vitamin E in reversing disease," says Blumberg. Yet the effects on younger and healthier individuals may be more promising.

Despite a substantial amount of research on vitamin E, Shibamoto advises that there is still much to learn—about how vitamin E works with other antioxidants and food components and, particularly, the optimal amount of vitamin E and other antioxidants for specific individuals that may produce favorable health outcomes.

Until more is known, Blumberg and Shibamoto agree with other experts who believe it may be premature to make sweeping recommendations about whether to supplement with vitamin E. Yet, Blumberg adds it is reasonable to suggest that the potential benefits of vitamin E seem to outweigh the risk (if any), especially for at-risk individuals. Studies suggesting greater risk with vitamin E supplements containing more than 400 IU observed no harm at lower levels, such as 100 IU per day.

The IFIC Foundation and Institute of Food Technologists (IFT) *Guidelines for Communicating the Emerging Science of Dietary Components for Health* suggest that consumers should be guided to make lifestyle changes based on consensus science, rather than emerging science. To do so, communicators are advised to:

- Convey emerging science on a continuum, based on the strength of the overall evidence as opposed to isolated studies

- Provide context when new or emerging scientific evidence adds to and supports the body of research currently available or when the emerging science contradicts previous research, questioning established dietary guidance

(For more information on the *Guidelines*, please visit the IFIC Foundation Web site at: http://www.ific.org/nutrition/functional/guidelines. For more information on how to critically review scientific studies, see the IFIC Review: *How to Understand and Interpret Food and Health-Related Scientific Studies* http://ific.org/publications/reviews/scientificir.cfm).

The latest findings pose some perplexing questions about vitamin E, but do not revoke the body of evidence that supports the safety and potential benefits of vitamin E supplements for a healthy population, as well as at-risk individuals, at the most common daily doses (100-400 IU) found in vitamin E supplements. One conclusion researchers can agree on: vitamin E, or any food component by itself, cannot match the most effective ways to reduce disease risk—not smoking, getting regular exercise, maintaining a healthy weight, and eating an overall health-ful diet.

Table 1.
Recommended Dietary Allowances for Vitamin E

Age (years)	RDA for Vitamin E (mg alpha-tocopherol)*
1-3	6 (9 IU)
4-8	7 (10.5 IU)
9-13	11 (16.5 IU)
14 +	15 (22.5 IU)
Pregnancy	15 (22.5 IU)
Lactation	19 (28.5 IU)

* 1 mg ATE vitamin E = 1.5 IU (ATE: alpha-tocopherol equivalents)

Source: Institute of Medicine, Food and Nutrition Board. Dietary Reference Intakes: Vitamin C, Vitamin E, Selenium, and Carotenoids. National Academy Press, 2000.

Related Information:

On the Web you'll find the IFIC Foundation and Institute of Food Technologists' (IFT) *Guidelines*
for Communicating the Emerging Science of Dietary Components for Health. The entire Guidelines are posted at: http://ific.org/nutrition/functional/guidelines/index.cfm

Also view the entire Guidelines at: http://ific.org/nutrition/functional/guidelines/guidelinesfulldoc.cfm.

Creating the Guidelines

According to the IFIC Foundation and IFT Web site at: http://ific.org/nutrition/functional/guidelines/guidelinesfulldoc.cfm, Journalism and nutrition professionals at Purdue University, University of Illinois, Urbana-Champaign, and University of Missouri, Columbia partnered on and assisted with the development of Guidelines for Communicating the Emerging Science of Dietary Components for Health. According to the Guideline Web site, the following challenges are presented to help the media communicate the health functions of foods and dietary supplements as reprinted with permission below.

The *Guidelines* are on the Web and accessible to the public also in a PDF file at: http://ific.org/nutrition/functional/guidelines/guidelinesfulldoc.cfm. According to the Web site, the role of the nutrition communicator is to empower consumers. The entire Guidelines' is 12 pages in length as a PDF file. The whole idea behind nutrition communication is, as is the summary in the Guidelines'PDF file states: "Scientific research is evolutionary, not revolutionary. Tell consumers where new findings fall on the research continuum and within the overall body of evidence."

According to the site, consumer communicators affect behavior by bridging the gap between scientist and consumer. Since the consumer rarely visits medical school libraries to read scientific journal articles, even though those libraries are open to the public, the consumer communicator has a specific role: to share meaning accurately. To communicate is to balance.

To develop the *Guidelines*, The International Food Information Council Foundation and the Institute of Food Technologists partnered with the faculty of the United States Department of Agriculture (USDA)/Initiative for Future Agriculture & Food Systems Research Program on Component Interactions for Functional Foods who provided time and expertise that has been instrumental in the development of the Guidelines.

If you're looking for resource material to develop into a topic, or if you're a journalist, librarian, teacher, public speaker, or student, here's where to start your research on how to communicate about food and health with the public. Physicians, nurses, genetic counselors, and nutrition professionals who also write or speak publicly also need to understand the role and behavior surrounding consumer communications.

What are the *Guidelines'* Main Goals?

Communicating the Health Functions of Foods & Dietary Supplements
A unique area of nutrition, dietary components for health, referred to commonly as "functional foods" or "bioactives for health," presents the following challenges:

- Empowering consumers to view beneficial dietary components as one part of a healthful diet and lifestyle rather than as "magic bullets."

- Balancing increased consumption of beneficial components within the proper caloric intake necessary to maintain a healthful weight.

- Communicating which segments of the population would likely benefit from increased or decreased consumption of a given component.

Communications about dietary components for health promotion hold promise to profoundly affect public knowledge, behavior, and well-being. Communicators have the opportunity to bridge the gap between science and the consumer by utilizing guidelines for translating research findings into understandable and actionable messages for consumers.

Guidelines for Communicating the Emerging Science of Dietary Components for Health

1. Enhance public understanding of foods, food components, and/or dietary supplements and their role in a healthful lifestyle.

2. Clearly convey the differences between emerging and consensus science.

3. Communicate with accuracy and balance.

4. Put new findings into the context needed for an individual to make dietary decisions.

5. Disclose all key details about a particular study.

6. Consider peer-review status.

7. Assess the objectivity of research.

(Harvard School of Public Health and IFIC Foundation, Improving Public Understanding: Guidelines for Communicating Emerging Science on Nutrition, Food Safety, and Health, 1998, http://ific. org/publications/brochures/guidelinesbroch.cfm). Communicators are challenged to:

• Convey emerging science on a continuum, based on the strength of the overall evidence, as opposed to isolated studies.

• Communicate the latest scientific findings with balance, while recognizing, but not overstating, differences of opinion.

• Provide context when new or emerging scientific evidence adds to and supports the body of research currently available or when the emerging science contradicts previous research, questioning established dietary guidance.

• Educate the public about a new area of research or technology, including complex terminology, before related nutrition information is likely to be understood.

APPENDIX A

Nutrition Time Lines

If you were to draw a timeline destined for daily newspapers today focusing on nutrition history, it would show a diagram of the ways in which science throughout the ages has been pitted against nature.

Below are some timelines on the Web, which include some nutrition milestones.

http://www.ars.usda.gov/is/timeline/nutrition.htm

http://www.ars.usda.gov/is/timeline/leg.htm

http://www.ars.usda.gov/is/search.
htm?btnG=Go%21&site=usda&ie=&output=xml_no_dtd&client=usda&as_site
search=http%3A%2F%2Fwww.ars.usda.gov%2Fis&http_referrer=http%253A
%252F%252Fwww%252Ears%252Eusda%252Egov%252Fis%252Fsearch%2
52Ehtm&q=nutrition+timeline&btnG=Go%21

Nutrition Time Line Needed in Mass Media

The left side of the time line would begin with the basic Paleolithic diet compared to the grain-based Neolithic diet—hunter/gatherer against farmer/herder. The diet of the farmer becomes different from the diet of the hunter/gather. Grains, breads, and fermented beverages largely replace fish, meat, nuts, seasonal fruits, nuts, wild vegetables, wild grass seeds, berries, and wild edible herbs. This is the beginning of how nature has been compared with technology.

The time line would look like this:
Paleolithic Diet.
Neolithic Diet.
Classical Mediterranean Diet.
Medieval Diet. Renaissance Diet.
Enlightenment Diet

Whole Grains-Based 19th Century Diet

20th Century Diet of Technology-Based Preserved Food—Heated Cereal—Convenience Food Diet with Added Sugar and "Evaporated Cane Juice" Added.

21st Century Obese Children's Diet of Soda, Chips, Fast Foods, Pizza, Burgers, Trans-Fats, and Sugary Snacks.

Nutrition Time Lines

If you were to draw a timeline destined for daily newspapers today focusing on nutrition history, it would show a diagram of the ways in which science throughout the ages has been pitted against nature. The left side of the time line would begin with the basic Paleolithic diet compared to the grain-based Neolithic diet—hunter/gatherer against farmer/herder.

The diet of the farmer becomes different from the diet of the hunter/gather. Grains, breads, and fermented beverages largely replace fish, meat, nuts, seasonal fruits, nuts, wild vegetables, wild grass seeds, berries, and wild edible herbs. This is the beginning of how nature has been compared with technology.

The time line would look like this:

Paleolithic Diet.

Neolithic Diet.

Classical Mediterranean Diet.

Medieval Diet. Renaissance Diet.

Enlightenment Diet

Whole Grains-Based 19th Century Diet

20th Century Diet of Technology-Based Preserved Food—Heated Cereal—Convenience Food Diet with Added Sugar and "Evaporated Cane Juice" Added.

21st Century Obese Children's Diet of Soda, Chips, Fast Foods, Pizza, Burgers, Trans-Fats, and Sugary Snacks.

Nutrition Timelines 1833-2000
History of Nutrition Time Line Before 1870

(Reprinted with the permission of the US Department of Agriculture, Agricultural Research Service; the in-house research arm of the USDA. The full time line can be seen online at: http://www.ars.usda.gov/is/timeline/1860chron.htm. Due to space limitations here, some time line entries from the original time line were not included. Check the Web site for the original time line.)

1833-1870

1833
Hog cholera first reported in the U.S.

1839
Library of the USDA established.

1843
Contagious bovine pleuropneumonia first introduced into the U.S.

1855—the first children's hospital is developed

1860
Farmers made up 58 percent of the labor force.

1860—Abraham Jacobi, MD begins formal courses in pediatrics and teaches infant nutrition

1861
Proved that *Phytophthora infestans* caused Irish potato famine.

1862
USDA created.

Morrill Land-Grant College Act authorized public land grants for colleges to teach agriculture and mechanic arts.

First USDA research bulletin issued, on sugar content of several varieties of grapes and their suitability for wine.

Homestead Act passed.

1863
First monthly crop report published by USDA.

Dry farming, as type of commercial agriculture, began in Utah.

1864
Pasteurization invented.

1866
Gregor Mendel showed that traits pass from parents to offspring, the foundation of modern genetics.

1867
Patrons of Husbandry, later known as the National Grange, organized by USDA employee. This was the first general farmers organization to permit women equality of membership and privilege.

1868
Division of Botany created to preserve herbarium material collected in government expeditions.

Refrigerator railroad car patented.

USDA began research on animal diseases.

1869
First analysis of food published in the U.S., for corn.

◆   ◆   ◆

Nutrition Time Line After 1870 to 1978

(Reprinted in part with permission from CHDD Media, University of Washington, Seattle, WA 98195-7920. The original timeline appeared in the University of Washington's LEND nutrition module and was adapted from an MCHB publication timeline.)

1872—the American Public Health Association is organized

1877—fourteen states have established state health agencies

1898—school lunches are introduced in New York City schools

1895—milk stations are established in New York City and Rochester (1897) to provide safe milk for infants and children and to educate parents about child hygiene and feeding

1897—services for crippled children (CCS) are initiated in Minnesota, and special schools for children who are deaf, blind, or mentally retarded are developed

1900-1909:

Municipal nursing services begin to develop, primarily in voluntary agencies such as Visiting Nurse Associations
  Organized prenatal care begins in Boston
  Pasteurized milk is introduced

1910-1919:

1915—The discovery of vitamins and the elucidation of their role exert a major influence on infant nutrition

1917—Frances Stern and Lucy Gillett are pioneers in community nutrition work in Boston

1918—The first nutrition publication, Milk the Indispensible Food for Children, is developed by the Children's Bureau and makes a plea for giving priority to infants and young children in allocating inadequate supplies

1920-1929:

1920—Nutrition studies of children in selected geographic areas of the nation are initiated by the Children's Bureau

1921-1929—The Sheppard-Towner Act is enacted and results in the development of full-time MCH units in the state health agencies. States give considerable attention to nutrition services and employ nutrition personnel

The Children's Bureau publishes height and weight tables for children under six years of age for use by health workers and issues a publication, Nutrition Work for Preschool Children, which provides one of the first descriptions of the activities of nutrition workers on behalf of preschool children
The American Child Health Association expands its scope of interest to include nutrition

1930-1939:

1930—Nutrition is a major concern of the 1930 White House Conference, which focuses on child growth and development

1935—Nationwide food consumption survey is initiated by the USDA

1935—Title V of the Social Security Act is passed and provides for three grant-in-aid programs, Maternal and Child Health, Crippled Children's Services, and Child Welfare. Nutrition positions are established in state health agencies and progressively increase in number as a result of the availability of Title V funds.

1936—The Children's Bureau employs its first nutrition consultant, Marjorie Heseltine. She provides national leadership and is a pioneer in the development of nutrition services in maternal and child health.

1939—Emergency relief and food assistance for people in need receive high priority, and the Food Stamp Program is created

1940-1949:

1940—The 4th White House Conference on Children addresses problems of nutrition and includes nutrition services among its recommendations

1941—The National Nutrition Conference results in the development of Recommended Dietary Allowances

1941—A second nutritionist, Helen Stacey, is added to the staff of the Children's Bureau.

1943—Graduate Training Programs in Public Health Nutrition are developed and Title V funds are made available for a nutrition training program

1946—The National School Lunch Program is established

1950-1959:

The Children's Bureau develops workshops on nutrition and diet in relation to mental retardation to upgrade the knowledge and skills of nutrition personnel in this area and provide a basis for the planning and development of nutrition services

The Indian Health Service, Public Health Service, establishes a nutrition unit to expand and improve nutrition services to Native Americans and Alaska natives

Nutrition Practices: A Guide for Public Health Administrators is published by the American Public Health Association

1960-1969:

1964—The Head Start Program is established and includes a nutrition component

1964—Dietary consultation services in states continue to expand (e.g., New Jersey surveys feeding practices in a sample of pediatric units of hospitals)

1966—The Child Nutrition Act is passed and expands food programs for children

1967—Title V funds support establishment of an intensive course in pediatric nutrition to upgrade knowledge and skills of nutrition practitioners

1968—Supplementary Food Programs for Low Income Groups Vulnerable to Malnutrition are initiated by the USDA

1970-1979:

1972—The Special Supplemental Food Program for Women, Infants, and Children (WIC) is established as an adjunct to health care

1977—The Nutrition Education and Training Program is established

1978—Guide for Developing Nutrition Services in Community Health Programs is published

1978—The Child Care Food Program becomes a permanent program and serves child care centers, settlement houses, recreation centers, institutions for the handicapped, and other group care facilities

USDA's Nutrition Timeline 1976-2000

(Reprinted with permission of the US Department of Agriculture (USDA). The timeline appears online at: http://www.ars.usda.gov/is/timeline/comp.htm.)

1976
SuperSlurper patented, a combination of starch and a synthetic chemical that absorbs hundreds of times its own weight in water.

Beef Research and Information Act passed.

Federal Land

Policy and Management Act repealed Homestead Act and many other land laws. Propagated bovine leukemia virus in cell culture.

Daws soft white winter wheat released; outstanding cold hardiness.

Citrus black fly eradicated using lab-reared parasites as biocontrol agents.

Designed, built, and operated a prototype system to continuously process raw cotton stock into yarn.

Crystalline sugar produced from sweet sorghum.

Atlantic potato released; number one Propagated chipping variety.

Controlled alligator weed in the southeastern U.S. using biological control.

Developed rapid, nondestructive technique for determining quality of forages used as feed for livestock, using near-infrared reflectance spectroscopy.

1977
Methods developed to determine exact sequence of DNA.

Demonstrated the stability of the transmissible mink encephalopathy agent.

Developed practice of spraying calcium chloride or calcium nitrate on unsprayed fruit to reduce blemishes.

Discovered direct relationship between *Neotyphodium coenophialum* fungus in fescue and disease in cattle.

1978
United States declared free of hog cholera Cryotherapy proved in treating malignant cancer in successful animals.

Developed technique to accurately measure vitamin D2 in plants, vitamin D3 in animals and their 11 metabolites.

1979
Smallpox eliminated, the only microbial disease ever completely defeated.

Sunburst tangerine released. 1980
Lactase enzymes evaluated; provided basis for lactose-reduced dairy products.

Supreme Court ruled that microbes created by genetic engineering could be patented.

Term "transgenic" coined to describe mice that carried a new, recently introduced gene.

NW-63 small red bean released; most widely grown small red cultivar in the U.S.

Discovered that peroxide dissolves lignin in crop residue so that the digestive bacteria in livestock can reach the cellulose fibers.

System developed to hold, transport, and deliver broilers and turkeys from the farm to the processing plant.

Developed vacuum infusion process by removing citrus peel from fresh fruit.

Stevenson-Wydler Technology Innovation Act passed.

CREAMS:A Field Scale Model for Chemicals, Runoff, and Erosion From Agricultural Management Systems published.

Eurasian pine adelgid in Hawaii controlled using biological control.

Marshall hard red spring wheat released.

Nosema locustae became the first protozoan registered as a microbial insecticide in the U.S.

1981
Foot-and-mouth disease vaccine developed; first effective subunit vaccine for any animal or human disease using gene splicing.

Isolated antitumor agent sesbanimide from coffee bean seeds.

Developed method for vaccinating chicks against Marek's disease through the eggshell, demonstrating for the first time that resistance to disease could be established by that method.

Determined that locoweed poisoning, in combination with high altitudes, could cause congestive heart failure in cattle.

Discovered plasmids that could be used to breed plants with desirable traits.

Cablegation developed; an automatic surface irrigation system that uses gravity to deliver water.

Columbia root-knot nematode discovered.

Lemhi Russet released; outyields Russet Burbank.

Developed techniques for the first commercial application of nematodes for control of carpenterworm in commercial fig orchards in California.

1982
New infectious agent, "prions," discovered; proposed as cause of transmissible spongiform encephalopathy diseases.

Genetically engineered human insulin produced.

First genetically engineered crop plant developed (tomato).

Developed the tree-banding technique used by homeowners to prevent gypsy moth caterpillars from crawling up tree trunks.

1983
Polymerase chain reaction devised; replicates large quantities of DNA from a small initial sample.

Discovered "jumping genes," or moveable genetic elements.

Lemont rice released; one of leading varieties grown in Texas, Mississippi, and Louisiana.

Controlled alfalfa blotch-leaf miner in the eastern U.S. using biological control.

1984
First transgenic farm animals born (sheep and pigs).

Tracheal mite found in honeybees.

Alginate gels and granules from seaweed used to encapsulate chemical or biological pesticides.

Bozoisky Russian wildrye released; dominant variety in the West.

Hycrest released; first interspecific hybrid of crested wheatgrass.

1985
Food Security Act established Conservation Reserve Program for highly erodible lands.

DNA fingerprinting invented.

Hole in Earth's ozone shield discovered over Antarctica.

Chester thornless blackberry released; predominant blackberry of its type in the world.

Discovered rubisco activase; protein responsible for action of rubisco.

Discovered that chemicals produced by aquatic microorganisms, geosmin and BIV, cause off-flavors in catfish.

1986
Germplasm Resources Information Network (GRIN) established; the world's most comprehensive database of agriculturally important plants.

Starch-encapsulation technique for pesticides developed.

Federal Technology Transfer Act passed.

First genetically engineered vaccine licensed by USDA, for pseudorabies in swine.

Synthesized pheromone from the papaya fruit fly as the first environmentally safe lure for females.

Discovered hormone PTTH that controls growth and molting in gypsy moth.

Discovered that pyrrolizidine alkaloids—natural chemicals found in hundreds of plants—kill livestock by causing cumulative and irreversible damage to the liver.

Isolated and characterized the structure of insect neuropeptides.

Othello pinto beans released; dominated acreage in the U.S. and Canada from 1988 to 1997.

Developed sunflower hybrids that produce oil several times higher in oleic acid than traditional sunflower oil; provided genetic material to industry to create NuSun hybrids.

Conducted studies that led to *Bacillus thuringiensis* registration as the first microbial insecticide for use on stored grain.

1987
Developed Fast Africanized Bee Identification System (FABIS) to distinguish European honeybees from Africanized honeybees.

First 100-percent soybean ink developed in four colors.

Released germplasm lines of sunflower with genetic resistance to all known races of downy mildew.

Developed microinjection technique to move a whole chromosome into a single cell of another plant.

Discovered that boron is a nutritionally necessary trace mineral.

Fallglo tangerine released; Sunburst and Fallglo comprise most of the early season tangerine market in Florida.

1988
Virus genes transferred to chickens to impart resistance to avian leukosis virus.

First authorized release of genetically altered bacteria outdoors.

Varroa mites found in Wisconsin.

First patent for genetically engineered animal issued.

Madsen soft white winter wheat released; first winter wheat variety in the U.S. with resistance to strawbreaker foot rot.

Discovered that lactose significantly reduced *Salmonella* bacteria in infected chickens.

Proved that antibiotics produced by soil bacteria responsible for take-all decline.

Developed anaplasma probe used to detect infected ticks.

Fortune plum released.

Sparkleberry holly released.

Created first relatively inexpensive and safe soil monolith collection procedure for 70+ milligram soil monoliths for lysimeters.

1890 Initiative by USDA

1989
Successfully separated living sperm into male- and female-producing batches.

Water Erosion Prediction Project model developed.

Waldo trailing blackberry released; first thornless trailing blackberry.

Identified a new parasite, *Neospora caninum*, as a cause of birth defects in cattle and sheep.

Isolated and cloned gene that triggers production of ACC synthase; modified gene to block ethylene production and delay ripening of tomatoes.

Ambersweet released; the first orange created by hybridization and selection.

Discovered the hormone that controls sex pheromone production in moths.

Bounty peach released.

Blackhawk black bean released; the first bean completely resistant to anthracnose.
1990

Oatrim fat replacer for food developed from soluble oat fiber and natural enzymes.

Food, Agriculture, Conservation, and Trade Act passed.

Technique developed to grow taxol-producing cells in tissue culture.

Nonindigenous Aquatic Nuisance Prevention and Control Act passed.

Africanized honeybees entered the U.S.

Demonstrated that genes could be infected using a commercially available inoculation device dubbed "gene gun"

Developed test to rapidly diagnose citrus blight. 1991

Rely soft white club wheat released; main club wheat cultivar in the U.S. since 1996.

Ranger Russet potato released.

Discovered first-ever homeobox—region of a gene that enables it to control other genes—in plants.

Patented new soybean inoculant—live, nitrogen-fixing bacteria—that increased soybean yield up to 2.9 bushels per acre.

Shasta viburnum released.

Diana hibiscus released.

1992
Entire sequence of one out of 16 chromosomes of a yeast identified.

Generated molecular probes to detect citrus canker disease.

SoilGardTM, the first commercial biocontrol agent for soil-borne diseases, developed in cooperation with industry.

Identified and cloned genes responsible for antibiotic production in soil bacteria responsible for take-all decline.

First sensitive and specific test for *Babesia equii* antibody developed.

Patented test to differentiate strains of citrus tristeza; a virus that can kill trees. Eskimo viburnum released.

Galaxy magnolia released.

1993
First genetic map of blueberry constructed.

Developed paper from chicken feathers.

Showed that deficiency in either selenium or vitamin E can trigger a mutation in a normal benign human virus; first report of a specific nutritional deficiency permitting a nonvirulent virus to become virulent.

Discovered that latex from guayule does not contain the allergens found in latex from the Brazilian rubber tree.

Potomac pear released.

Developed remote-sensing technology to measure surface soil moisture, temperature, and other landscape characteristics.

1994
Fantesk invented; an inseparable mixture of starch and oil.

Oxygen Radical Absorbance Capacity (ORAC) method of measuring antioxidant capacity automated.

Developed method to genetically modify *Brucella abortus* Strain 19, to differentiate between naturally infected and vaccinated animals.

First genetic linkage maps of cattle and swine constructed.

First sensitive and specific test developed for malignant catharrhal fever in sheep.

Black emerald grapes released.

1995
First complete genome sequence of a microorganism described.

Little Giant processing blueberry released.

Conducted extensive outdoor tests with PAM, polyacrylamide powder, showing its efficacy in preventing irrigation water from carrying away soil particles as the water flows down a furrow and leading to widespread use.

First two postharvest biofungicides registered with EPA—ASPIRE and BIO-SAVE 11—based on ARS research.

Revised Universal Soil Loss Equation completed. Valley Forge and New Harmony elm trees released; tolerant to Dutch elm disease.

Experimentally infected cattle with transmissible mink encephalopathy and scrapie agents.

Dwelley, Sanford, and Myles chickpeas released; resistant to ascochyta blight.

1996
Federal Agriculture Improvement and Reform Act passed.

Amendments to the Safe Drinking Water Act passed.

Isolated and developed DNA test to identify bacterium that caused swine diarrhea.

First sensitive and specific test for anaplasmosis antibody in cattle developed.

1997
Cloned a plant-derived gene for resistance to a plant virus, the "N" gene.

"Dolly" cloned from an udder cell of an adult sheep.

Phytoplasma discovered as the infectious cause of commercially desirable free-branching growth habit in poinsettia.

Developed technique for large-scale extraction of limonoid glucosides from citrus. Trailblazer alfalfa released.

1998
Bacterial microbe mixture PREEMPT developed for competitive exclusion of *Salmonella*.

Method developed to recycle chromium-containing solid waste from leather production.

First genetically engineered vaccine for shipping fever in cattle developed.

First effective lure for German yellowjacket and golden paper wasps developed.

Discovered that dogs are a definitive host for Neospora.

First sensitive and specific test to detect *Babesia caballi* antibody in horses developed.

Gene-based test for Johne's disease in cattle developed.

Bluebyrd plum released.

1999
Executive Order 13112 on Invasive Species signed.

Modified live-bacterium fish vaccine approved; protects young channel catfish against enteric septicemia.

2000
First DNA sequencing of a plant genome, the flowering mustard *Arabidopsis thaliana*. ARS one of a three-member U.S. team.

Pierce's disease first discovered in U.S.

First cloned transgenic animal produced that carries a gene designed to enhance the health and well-being of the animal. This cow has the potential to produce an enzyme that destroys mastitis-causing bacteria.

Nutrim, obtained from the thermo-mechanical processing of oats, developed and patented as a commercial soluble oat fiber nutraceutical.

First pathogenic bacterium identified that does not need or use iron. The bacterium causes Lyme disease in humans.

Demonstrated that pure prion proteins can trigger normal proteins to change shape and become infectious.

Molecular technique developed that will enable researchers to induce mutations in the Marek's disease herpesvirus genome, called overlapping cosmid clone library (OCCL).

First soybeans with complete nematode resistance developed.

The major human allergen in soybean seed suppressed by sequence-mediated gene silencing in transgenic soybeans.

Green Dixie, the first green blackeye-type southernpea, released.

Biomass Research and Development Act.

ARS-imported Russian honey bees transferred to the U.S. honey bee industry, resulting in honey bees resistant to parasitic mites.

Food Safety Initiative, modified food safety inspections to decrease foodborne illnesses.

Chemicals that induce an otherwise healthy plant to form a tumor to resist infection—called bruchins—discovered.

First molecular map of the ribosome, the cell's essential protein factory, completed.

APPENDIX B

Bibliography

Highly Recommended Books and Articles

Nutrition: Concepts and Controversies (with Nutrition Connections CD-ROM and InfoTrac) (Paperback) by Frances Sizer, Ellie Whitney. Brooks Cole;10 edition (May 2005).

Understanding Nutrition (with CD-ROM and InfoTrac) (Understanding Nutrition) by Eleanor Noss Whitney, Sharon Rady Rolfes (Hardcover—May 2004)

Study Guide for Whitney and Rolfes: Understanding Nutrition (Paperback) 2002.

Cecil Textbook of Medicine, 21st ed. W. B. Saunders Company; 2000.

Primary Care Medicine, 4th ed. Lippincott Williams & Wilkins; 2000.

The Holistic Cookbook, Renders, Eileen, N.D. Renders Publishing, 2001.

Noni Juice: How Much, How Often, For What, 3rd Edition
by Neil Solomon, MD, PhD 2000).

Cliver, D. O. and Newman, R. A. (eds.). 1984. *Drinking water microbiology.* NATO/CCMS Drinking Water Pilot Project Series (CCMS 128), Committee on the Challenges of Modern Society. Published by the US Environmental Protection Agency, Office of Drinking Water, Washington, DC 20460 (EPA 570/9 84 006), xxxii+545pp.

Cliver, D. O. and Cochrane, B. A. (eds.). 1986. *Progress in food safety.* Proceedings of a symposium entitled *"Progress in Our Knowledge of Foodborne Disease During the Life of the Food Research Institute,"* held 28 May 1986 at the University of Wisconsin Madison. Food Research Institute, University of Wisconsin Madison, vii+120 pp.

Cliver, D. O. (ed.). 1990. *Foodborne diseases.* Academic Press, San Diego. xvii+395 pp.

Hui, Y. H., J. R. Gorham, K. D. Murrell, and D. O. Cliver (eds.). 1994. *Foodborne Disease Handbook (in Three Volumes),* Marcel Dekker, New York. 2016 pp.

Cliver, D. O. 2000. Foodborne Diseases, 1st ed., Arabic translation. Scientific Publishing and Printing. King Saud's University, Riyadh, Arabic Kingdom of Saudi. ISBN: 9960-37-317-7

Cliver, D. O., and Riemann, H. P., eds. 2002. *Foodborne Diseases, 2d ed.,* Academic Press, London. xvii+407 pp.

Cotruvo, J. A., A. Dufour, G. Rees, J. Bartram, R. Carr, D. O. Cliver, G. F. Craun, R. Fayer and V. P. J. Gannon, eds. 2004. *Waterborne Zoonoses: Identification, Causes and Control.* IWA (International Water Association) Publishing, London. xvii + 506 pp.

Riemann, H. P., and Cliver, D. O., eds. 2005. *Foodborne Infections and Intoxications,* 3d ed., Academic Press, London, in press. (>900 pp.)

APPENDIX C

Associations

Associations of Interest to Nutritionists, Dieticians, and Health Care Professionals

American Dietetic Association
http://www.eatright.org

American Obesity Association
http://www.obesity.org

American Society for Nutritional Sciences
http://www.asns.org/

American Society for Clinical Nutrition
http://www.ascn.org/

The Annapolis Center for Science-Based Public Policy
http://www.annapoliscenter.org

Association of Food & Drug Officials
http://www.afdo.org

American Diabetes Association
http://www.diabetes.org

American Farm Bureau Federation
http://www.fb.com

American Heart Association
http://www.americanheart.org

Botanical Center for Age-Related Diseases
http://nccam.nih.gov/news/2005/040705.htm

Calorie Control Council
http://www.caloriecontrol.org

Center for Health Promotion
http://pan.ilsi.org

Consumer Healthcare Products Association
http://www.caloriecontrol.org

CropLife America
http://www.croplifeamerica.org

Egg Nutrition Center
http://www.enc-online.org

Food Marketing Institute
http://www.fmi.org

Food Allergy Research and Resource Program
http://www.farrp.org

Grocery Manufacturers of America
http://www.gmabrands.com

International Association for Food Protection
http://www.foodprotection.org

National Dairy Council/Dairy Management
http://www.dairyinfo.com

National Policy and Resource Center on Nutrition and Aging
http://www.fiu.edu/~nutreldr

North American Agricultural Journalists
http://naaj.tamu.edu/

Society for Nutrition Education
http://www.sne.org

World Sugar Research Organization
http://www.wsro.org

Government-Related Agencies

Centers for Disease Control and Prevention
http://www.cdc.gov

Center for Food Safety and Applied Nutrition
http://www.crfsan.fda.gov

Fight BAC™
http://www.fightbck.org

Food and Drug Administration: Consumer Inquiries
http://www.fda.gov

Joint Institute for Food Safety and Applied Nutrition
http://www.jifsan.umd.edu

National Cancer Institute: Press Office
http://www.nci.nih.gov

National Digestive Disease Information Clearinghouse
http://www.niddk.nih.gov

National Diabetes Information Clearinghouse
http://www.niddk.ninh.gov

National Health Information Center
http://health.gov/NHIC

National Institutes of Health
http://www.nih.gov

National Marine Fisheries Service
http://www.nmfs.noaa.gov

President's Council on Physical Fitness and Sports
http://fitness.gov

US Dept. of Agriculture
http://www.usda.gov

USDA/Food, Nutrition, and Consumer Services
http://www.fns.usda.gov/fncs

USDA/ Food Safety and Inspection Service Information
http://www.fsis.usda.gov

USDA/Meat and Poultry Hotline
Phone 1-800-535-4555

USDA/Animal and Plant Health Inspection Service
http://www.aphis.usda.gov

USDA/Foreign Agricultural Service
http://www.fas.usda.gov

USDA/National Agricultural Library
http://www.nalusda.gov

USDA/National Agriculture Statistics Service
http://www.fas.usda.gov

US Department of Health and Human Services
http://www.hhs.gov

Foodborne Illness Education Information Center
http://www.nalusda.gov/foodborne/index.html

US Department of Health and Human Services
http://www.hhs.gov

US Environmental Protection Agency
http://www.epa.gov

US Federal Trade Commission
http://www.ftc.gov

◆   ◆   ◆

Associations of Interest to Nutrition Journalists, Consumer Communications Professionals, and Medical or Science Journalists

American Medical Writers Association
40 West Gude Drive, Suite 101
Rockville, MD 20850-1192
http://www.amwa.org/default.asp?ID=1

American Society of Indexers (for indexing careers)
10200 West 44th Avenue, Suite 304,
Wheat Ridge, CO 80033
http://www.asindexing.org/site/index.html

American Society of Journalists and Authors
1501 Broadway, Suite 302
New York, NY 10036
http://www.asja.org

Association of Health Care Journalists (AHCJ)
Center for Excellence in Health Care Journalism
Missouri School of Journalism
10 Neff Hall
Columbia, MO 62511
http://www.ahcj.umn.edu/

Association of Professional Writing Consultants
http://www.consultingsuccess.org/index.htm

Council of Biology Editors
http://www.monroecc.edu/depts/library/cbe.htm

Council of the Advancement of Science Writing
P.O. Box 910
Hedgesville, WV 25427
http://www.casw.org/
Careers in Science Writing:
http://www.casw.org/careers.htm

Education Writers Association
2122 P Street, NW Suite 201
Washington, DC 20037
http://www.ewa.org/

International Food, Wine & Travel Writers Association (IFW&TWA)
1142 South Diamond Bar Boulevard #177
Diamond Bar, CA 91765-2203
http://www.ifwtwa.org/index.html

Journalism.org—Researches, Resources & Ideas to Improve Journalism
http://www.journalism.org/

National Association of
Science Writers, Inc.
P.O. Box 890, Hedgesville, WV 25427
http://www.nasw.org/

North American Agricultural Journalists
http://naaj.tamu.edu/

Society of Professional Journalists
Eugene S. Pulliam National Journalism Center
3909 N. Meridian St., Indianapolis, IN 46208
http://www.spj.org/

Society for Technical Communication
http://www.stc.org/

Text and Academic Authors Association
TAA
P.O. Box 76477
St. Petersburg, FL
http://www.taaonline.net/

World Association of Medical Editors
http://www.wame.org/
http://www.wame.org/index.htm

Diversified Media Associations of Interest to all Communicators

American Business Press
http://www.americanbusinesspress.com/

American Society of Business Press Editors
http://www.asbpe.org/

Associated Business Writers of America
http://www.poewar.com/articles/associations.htm

Associazioni ed Enti Professionali—America
http://www.alice.it/writers/grp.wri/wgrpame.htm
Contains a list of South American, Canadian, and US writers' organizations, including language translation firms.

American Marketing Association
http://www.marketingpower.com/content1539.php

Association of Professional Communications Consultants
http://www.consultingsuccess.org/index.htm

Writer's Encyclopedia A-Z List
WritersMarket.com
http://www.writersmarket.com/encyc/azlist.asp

Editorial Freelancers Association
http://www.the-efa.org/

Editor's Guild
http://www.edsguild.org/become.htm
The current online Yellow Pages, published annually since 1997 includes listings by skills as well as a specialties index. This association published the hardcopy, Yellow Pages, a listing of Association members who wished to advertise their skills and specialties, between 1989 and 1999.
http://www.tiac.net/users/freelanc/YP.html

International Women's Writing Guild
http://www.iwwg.com/index.php, Or: http://www.iwwg.com

The International Women's Writing Guild, headquartered in New York and founded in 1976, is a network for the personal and professional empowerment of women through writing.

Video Software Dealers Association
http://www.vsda.org/Resource.phx/vsda/index.htx

Public Relations Society of America
http://www.prsa.org/

Deep Dish TV
http://www.deepdishtv.org/pages/catalogue13.htm

Video History Project
http://www.experimentaltvcenter.org/history/groups/gtext.php3?id=37

Advertising Research Foundation
http://www.arfsite.org/

The Mail Preference Service
http://www.dmaconsumers.org/offmailinglist.html

Advertising Associations Directory
http://paintedcows.com/associations.html

Mailing Fulfillment Service Association
http://www.mfsanet.org/pages/index.cfm?pageid=1

Television Bureau of Advertising
http://www.tvb.org/nav/build_frameset.asp?url=/docs/homepage.asp

Home Improvement Research Institute
http://www.hiri.org/abouthiri.htm

Writers-Editors Network
http://www.writers-editors.com/

Professional and Technical Consultants Association
http://www.patca.org/html/articles/ratesurvey/ratesurvey1.htm

Association of Independent Commercial Producers
http://www.aicp.com/splash-noswf.html

National Cable & Telecommunications Association
http://www.ncta.com/

International Association of Women in Radio and Television
http://www.iawrt.org/

National Communication Association
http://www.natcom.org/nca/Template2.asp

The Association for Women in Communications
http://www.womcom.org/

Society of Telecommunications Consultants
http://www.stcconsultants.org/

European Training Media Association
http://www.etma.org/

Advertising Research Foundation
641 Lexington Avenue • New York, NY 10022
http://www.arfsite.org/

International Women's Media Foundation
http://www.iwmf.org/training/womensmedia.php

Independent Publishers Group
http://www.ipgbook.com/index.cfm?userid=36155756

American Society of Media Photographers
150 North Second Street, Philadelphia, PA 19106
(Electronic imaging and digital technology)
http://www.asmp.org/

International Interactive Communications Society
http://users.rcn.com/sfiics/

International Multimedia Association
http://www.emmac.org/

National Cable Television Association
http://www.museum.
tv/archives/etv/N/htmlN/nationalcabl/nationalcabl.htm

Information Technology Association of America
http://www.itaa.org/eweb/StartPage.aspx

Personal and Oral History Associations

Association of Personal Historians
http://www.personalhistorians.org/index.html

Oral History Association
http://omega.dickinson.edu/organizations/oha/about.html

International Oral History Association
http://www.ioha.fgv.br/ioha/english/index.html

Texas Oral History Association
http://www.baylor.edu/TOHA/

Southwest Oral History Association
http://soha.fullerton.edu/

New England Association for Oral History
http://www.ucc.uconn.edu/~cohadm01/neaoh.html

Michigan Oral History Association
http://www.umich.edu/pres/history/oral.html

UCLA Oral History Program
http://www.library.ucla.edu/libraries/special/ohp/ohpindex.htm

"California As I Saw It," First Person Narratives of California's Early Years:
1849-1900. The Library of Congress.
http://memory.loc.gov/ammem/cbhtml/cbhome.html

◆   ◆   ◆

Nutrition and Health-Related Associations, Research Institutes, Corporations, Academies, and University Programs

American Academy of Family Physicians: http://www.aafp.org/
American Association of Family and Consumer Sciences: http://www.aafcs.org/
American Dietetic Association: http://www.eatright.org/
American Heart Association: http://www.americanheart.org/
American Institute for Cancer Research: http://www.aicr.org/
American Public Health Association: http://www.apha.org/
American Society of Clinical Nutrition: http://www.ascn.org/
Center for Science in the Public Interest: http:// www.cspinet.org/
Chocolate Manufacturers Association: http://www.chocolateusa.org/
Consumer Federation of America: http://www.consumerfed.org/
Consumer Healthcare Products Association: http://www.chpa-info.org/
Council for Responsible Nutrition: http://www.crnusa.org/
Egg Nutrition Center: http://www.enc-online.org/
Federal Trade Commission: http://www.ftc.gov/
Food and Nutrition Board, Institute of Medicine: http://www.iom.edu/board.asp?id=3788
Foundation for American Communications: http://www.facsnet.org/
Asian Food Information Center: http://www.afic.org/Press%20Centre.htm
Institute of Food Technologists: http://www.ift.org/cms/
International Dairy Foods Association: http://www.idfa.org/
International Life Sciences Institute: http://www.ilsi.org/
Kleinfeld Kaplan & Becker: http://www.fda.gov/ohrms/dockets/dailys/00/Aug00/082400/cp0001.pdf
Lehigh University, Department of Journalism and Communication: http://www.lehigh.edu/~injrl/sciwrit/
National Cancer Institute, US National Institutes of Health: http://www.cancer.gov/

National Cooperative Business Association: http://www.ncba.coop/

National Food Processors Association: http://www.worldfooddayusa.org/CMS/2951/8939.aspx

National Potato Promotion Board: http://www.uspotatoes.com/ Office of Dietary Supplements, National Institutes of Health: http://ods.od.nih.gov/

The Popcorn Board: http://www.popcorn.org/index.cfm

Purdue University, National Institutes of Health Botanicals Center for Age-Related Diseases: http://www.purdue.edu/UNS/html4ever/000920.Weaver.nihcenter.html

Purdue University, Department of Foods and Nutrition: http://www.cfs.purdue.edu/

Rutgers University, Nutraceuticals Institute: http://foodsci.rutgers.edu/nci/

Soyfoods Association of North America: http://www.soyfoods.org/

Saint Joseph's University, Erivan K. Haub School of Business: http://www.sju.edu/

Tufts School of Medicine and Nutrition: http://www.tufts.edu/med/nutrition-infection/

Tufts University Health and Nutrition Letter: http://healthletter.tufts.edu/

United Soybean Board: http://www.unitedsoybean.org/

United States Department of Agriculture, Agricultural Research Service: http://www.ars.usda.gov/main/main.htm

United States Food and Drug Administration, Center for Food Safety and Applied Nutrition: http://www.cfsan.fda.gov/list.html

University of California, Davis: http://www.ucdavis.edu/index.html

University of California, Davis, California Institute of Food and Agricultural Research: http://aic.ucdavis.edu/

University of California, Davis, Robert Mondavi Institute for Wine and Food Science: http://www.news.ucdavis.edu/mondavi/iwfs_facts.html

University of Illinois, Department of Food Science and Human Nutrition: http://www.fshn.uiuc.edu/

University of Illinois, Functional Foods for Health Program: http://www.ag.uiuc.edu/~ffh/ffh.html

University of Massachusetts, Department of Food Science: http://www.umass.edu/foodsci/

University of Missouri, Columbia, Department of Food Science and Human Nutrition: http://outreach.missouri.edu/hes/food.htm

University of Missouri, Columbia, Missouri School of Journalism: http://journalism.missouri.edu/

University of Southern California, School of Pharmacy: http://www.usc.edu/schools/pharmacy/

Virginia Tech Center for Food and Nutrition Policy: http://www.vt.edu/ Food Safety Research Information Office: http://www.nal.usda.gov/fsrio/acad.htm

APPENDIX D

Resources (General)

American Dietetic Association
http://www.webdietitians.org/Public/

American Dietetic Association Evidence Analysis Library
http://www.adaevidencelibrary.org/default.cfm?
The ADA Evidence Analysis Library summarizes the best available research on dietetics and nutrition. To enter the library, choose one of the tabs (Diseases & Conditions, Nutrition Care, Food, Nutrients, or Contributors) in the menu at the top of the Evidence Analysis Library's Web site.

National Institute of Diabetes and Digestive and Kidney Diseases, Clinical Research Studies: http://clinicalstudies.info.nih.gov/cgi/protinstitute.cgi?NIDDK.0.html

National Diabetes Information Clearinghouse: http://diabetes.niddk.nih.gov/

School Nutrition Association: http://www.asfsa.org/

House Bill Addresses Food Allergies in Schools: http://www.asfsa.org/Index.aspx?id=1673

K-12 Health: Preventive Care and Nutrition: http://www.kidsource.com/kidsource/pages/k12.prevent.html

Vegetarian Nutrition for Teenagers: The Vegetarian Resource Group http://www.vrg.org/nutrition/teennutrition.htm

Cooking Schools & Catering: http://www.vrg.org/links/#schools

The Vegetarian Channel: http://www.thevegetarianchannel.com/

International Vegetarian Union: http://www.ivu.org/recipes/

Food & Beverage Network: http://www.foodandbeverage-network.com/

Cooperative Grocers' Information Network: http://www.cgin.coop/

Author's Web site: http://www.newswriting.net

Appendix E

Glossary

Glossary of Food-Related Terms

Aa

acceptable daily intake (ADI)—

The amount of chemical that, if ingested daily over a lifetime, appears to be without appreciable effect.

acesulfame K—

Acesulfame K, or acesulfame potassium, is a low-calorie sweetener approved for use in the United States in 1988. It is an organic salt consisting of carbon, nitrogen, oxygen, hydrogen, sulphur and potassium atoms. It is 200 times sweeter than sucrose, has a synergistic sweetening effect with other sweeteners, has a stable shelf-life and is heat stable. It is excreted through the human digestive system unchanged, and is therefore non-caloric.

additives (food additives)—

Any natural or synthetic material, other than the basic raw ingredients, used in the production of a food item to enhance the final product. Any substance that may affect the characteristics of any food, including those used in the production, processing, treatment, packaging, transportation or storage of food.

Adverse Reaction Monitoring System (ARMS)—

A system operated by FDA which monitors and investigates all complaints by individuals or their physicians that are believed to be related to a specific food, food and color additives or vitamin and mineral supplements. The ARMS computerized database helps officials decide whether reported adverse reactions represent a real public health risk associated with food so that appropriate action can be taken.

aerobic exercise—

Aerobic exercise refers to the kind of fast-paced activity that makes you "huff and puff." It places demands on your cardiovascular apparatus and, over time, produces beneficial changes in your respiratory and circulatory systems.

agrochemicals—

Term for artificially produced chemicals (such as feed additives, pharmaceuticals, fertilizers or pesticides) used in agriculture to improve crops or livestack production.

algin—

A compound which is extracted from algae and used in puddings, milk shakes and ice cream to make these foods creamier and thicker and to extend shelf life.

alitame—

A sweetener made from amino acids (L-aspartic acid, D-alanine, and a novel amide [a specific arrangement of chemical bonds between carbon, nitrogen and oxygen]). It offers a taste that is 2000 times sweeter than that of sucrose and can be used in a wide variety of products including beverages, tabletop sweeteners, frozen desserts and baked goods. Only the aspartic acid component of alitame is metabolized by the body. As a result, alitame contains 1.4 kcal/g. Since alitame is such an intense sweetener, however, it is used at very low levels and thus contributes negligible amounts of calories. It is highly stable, can withstand high temperatures in cooking and baking, and has the potential to be used in almost all foods and beverages in which sweeteners are presently used. FDA is currently considering a petition to approve its use in the United States food supply. Alitame has been approved for use in all food and beverage products in Australia, Mexico and New Zealand.

allergen (food allergen)—

A food allergen is the part of a food (a protein) that stimulates the immune system of food allergic individuals. A single food can contain multiple food allergens. Carbohydrates or fats are not allergens.

allergy (food allergy)—

A food allergy is any adverse reaction to an otherwise harmless food or food component (a protein) that involves the body's immune system. To avoid confusion with other types of adverse reactions to foods, it is important to use the terms "food allergy" or "food hypersensitivity" only when the immune system is involved in causing the reaction.

ally methyl trisulfide, dithiolthiones—

A type of sulfide/thiol found in cruciferous vegetables which may provide the health benefits of lowering LDL cholesterol and of maintaining a healthy immune system.

alpha-carotene—

A type of carotenoid found in carrots which provides the health benefit of neutralizing free radicals that may cause damage to cells.

alternative agriculture—

A range of technological and management option farms striving to reduce costs, protect health and environmental quality, and enhance beneficial biological interactions and natural processes. Alternative agriculture techniques cannot be uniformly applied across all commodities or all regions of the country. Such practices typically require more information, trained labor, time and management skills per unit of production than conventional farming.

Alzheimer's disease—

This disease causes progressive memory loss and dementia in its victims as it kills brain cells (neurons). It is named after Alois Alzheimer who in 1906 first described the Amyloid β Protein (AβP) plaques in the human brain that are caused by this disease. The drug Tacrine appears to slow the progression of Alzheimer's disease, but there is currently no way to stop the disease.

amino acids—

Amino acids function as the building blocks of proteins. Chemically, amino acids are organic compounds containing an amino (NH2) group and a carboxyl (COOH) group. Amino acids are classified as essential, nonessential and conditionally essential. If body synthesis is inadequate to meet metabolic need, an amino acid is classified as essential and must be supplied as part of the diet. Essential amino acids include leucine, isoleucine, valine, tryptophan, phenylalanine, methionine, threonine, lysine, histidine and possibly arginine. Nonessential amino acids can be synthesized by the body in adequate amounts, and include alanine, aspartic acid, asparagine, glutamic acid, glutamine, glycine, proline and serine. Conditionally essential amino acids become essential under certain clinical conditions.

anaphylaxis—

A rare but potentially fatal condition in which several different parts of the body experience food-allergic reactions simultaneously, causing hives, swelling of the throat and difficulty breathing. It is the most severe allergic reaction to an allergen and requires immediate medical attention when it occurs.

anemia—

Anemia is a condition in which a deficiency in the size or number of erythrocytes (red blood cells) or the amount of hemoglobin they contain limits the exchange of oxygen and carbon dioxide between the blood and the tissue cells. Most anemias are caused by a lack of nutrients required for normal erythrocyte synthesis, principally iron, vitamin B-12, and folic acid. Others result from a variety of conditions, such as hemorrhage, genetic abnormalities, chronic disease states or drug toxicity.

Animal and Plant Health Inspection Service (APHIS)—

A government agency which resides in the United States Department of Agriculture and governs the field-testing of agricultural biotechnology crops.

Anorexia Nervosa—

An eating disorder characterized by refusal to maintain a minimally normal weight for height and age. The condition includes weight loss leading to maintenance of body weight 15 percent below normal; an intense fear of weight gain or becoming fat, despite the individual's underweight status; a disturbance in the self-awareness of one's own body weight or shape; and in females, the absence of at least three consecutive menstrual cycles that would otherwise be expected to occur.

anthocyanidins—

A type of flavonoid found in various fruits which provides the health benefits of neutralizing free radicals and possibly reducing the risk of cancer.

antibiotic resistance—

The ability of a bacterium to synthesize a protein that neutralizes an antibiotic.

antibiotics—

Antibiotics are used in animal agriculture for two reasons. First, to improve the rate of growth and the feed efficiency of animals so they produce more meat or milk on less feed. The second reason is to prevent and treat diseases, just as in humans.

antibody—

Protein produced by the immune system of humans and higher animals in response to the presence of a specific antigen.

anticarcinogens—

Substances which inhibit the formation of cancers or the growth of tumors. More than 600 chemicals are claimed to be anti-cancer agents. These range from natural chemical constituent present in garlic, broccoli, cabbage and green tea to manmade antioxidants, such as butylated hydroxyanisole (BHA) and derivatives of retinoic acid.

antigen—

A foreign substance (almost always a protein) that, when introduced into the body, stimulates an immune response.

antioxidant—

Antioxidants protect key cell components by neutralizing the damaging effects of "free radicals," natural byproducts of cell metabolism. Free radicals form when oxygen is metabolized, or burned by the body. They travel through cells, disrupting the structure of other molecules, causing cellular damage. Such cell damage is believed to contribute to aging and various health problems.

antisense—

A piece of DNA that produces the mirror image, or antisense messenger RNA, that is exactly opposite in sequence to one that directs the cells to produce a specific protein. Since the antisense RNA binds tightly to its image, it prevents the protein from being made.

ascorbic acid—

Also known as vitamin C, it is essential for the development and maintenance of connective tissue. Vitamin C speeds the production of new cells in wound healing and it is an antioxidant that keeps free radicals from hooking up with other molecules to form damaging compounds that might attack tissue. Vitamin C protects the immune system, helps fight off infections, reduces the severity of allergic reactions and plays a role in the synthesis of hormones and other body chemicals. Green peppers, broccoli, citrus fruits, tomatoes, strawberries, and other fresh fruits and vegetables are good sources of vitamin C.

aspartame—

Aspartame is a low-calorie sweetener used in a variety of foods and beverages and as a tabletop sweetener. It is about 200 times sweeter than sugar. Aspartame is made by joining two protein components, aspartic acid and phenylalanine.

asthma—

Asthma is a chronic medical condition, affecting approximately 10 million Americans (3 to 4 percent of the population). Asthma results when irritants (or trigger substances) cause swelling of the tissues in the air passage of the lungs, making it difficult to breathe. Typical symptoms of asthma include wheezing, shortness of breath and coughing.

atherosclerosis—

A condition that exists when too much cholesterol builds up in the blood and accumulates in the walls of the blood vessels.

Attention Deficit Hyperactivity Disorder (ADHD)—

Commonly called "hyperactivity," Attention Deficit Hyperactivity Disorder is a clinical diagnosis based on specific criteria. These include excessive motor activity, impulsiveness, short attention span, low tolerance to frustration and onset before 7 years of age.

Back to top

Bb

basal metabolism—

Basal metabolism is the energy (calories) a body burns when completely at rest. Basal metabolism rate (BMR) is the level of energy needed to keep involuntary body processes going. These processes include heartbeat, breathing, generating body heat, perspiring to keep cool, and transmitting messages to the brain. For a sedentary person, BMR accounts for about 60-70 percent of daily energy expenditure; the remaining 30-40 percent is from physical activity and from body heat produced after a meal. Physical activity is responsible for as much as 50-60 percent of the total energy expenditure in people who include frequent aerobic activity into their lifestyles

basophils—

Blood cells which when connected to immunoglobulin E antibodies release histamine or other substances causing allergic symptoms.

beta-carotene—

A type of carotenoid found in various fruits and vegetables which provide the health benefit of neutralizing free radicals that may cause damage to cells.

beta glucan—

A soluble fiber in oats which provides the health benefit of reducing the risk of cardiovascular disease by decreasing circulating blood cholesterol.

bias—

Bias occurs when problems in study design lead to effects that are not related to the variables being studied. An example is selection bias, which occurs when study subjects are chosen in a way that can misleadingly increase or decrease the strength of an association. Choosing experimental and control group subjects from different populations would result in a selection bias.

biodegradable—

Describes any material that can be broken down by biological action (e.g., dissimilation, digestion, denitrification). The breakdown of material (chemicals) by microorganisms (bacteria, fungus, etc.).

biological activity—

The effect (change in metabolic activity upon living cells) caused by specific compounds or agents. For example, the drug aspirin causes the blood to thin, that is to clot less easily.

biological controls—

An integrated pest management method which includes the use of living organisms to reduce the extent of pest problems. This includes the use of beneficial or predatory insects such as ladybugs and parasitic wasps to control crop-destroying bugs.

biopesticide—

A biopesticide is any material of natural origin used in pest control derived from living organisms, such as bacteria, plant cells or animal cells.

biotechnology—

The simplest definition of biotechnology is "applied biology." The application of biological knowledge and techniques to develop products. It may be further defined as the use of living organisms to make a product or run a process. By this definition, the classic techniques used for plant and animal breeding, fermentation and enzyme purification would be considered biotechnology. Some people use the term only to refer to newer tools of genetic science. In this context, biotechnology may be defined as the use of biotechnical methods to modify the genetic materials of living cells so they will produce new substances or perform new functions. Examples include recombinant DNA technology, in which a copy of a piece of DNA containing one or a few genes is transferred between organisms or "recombined" within an organism.

blind (single or double) experiment—

In a single blind experiment, the subjects do not know whether they are receiving an experimental treatment or a placebo. In a double blind experiment, neither the researchers nor the participants are aware of which subjects receive the treatment—until after the study is completed.

body mass index (BMI)—

Method used for determining overweight and obesity in adults. BMI is a calculation that divides a person's weight in kilograms by height in meters squared (BMI = $[kg/m^2]$). BMI can also be calculated in pounds and inches: BMI=$[lbs/in^2]$ X 703. The general guideline currently recommended by the Center for Disease Control and Prevention is that individuals with a BMI of 25 to 29.9 are considered overweight and those individuals with a BMI greater than 30 are considered obese.

Bovine spongiform encephalopathy (BSE)—

Bovine spongiform encephalopathy, or BSE, is also known as "mad cow disease." It is a rare, chronic degenerative disease affecting the brain and central nervous system of cattle. Cattle with BSE lose their coordination, develop abnormal posture and experience changes in behavior. Clinical symptoms take 4-5 years to develop, followed by death in a period of several weeks to months unless the affected animal is destroyed sooner.

rBST (bovine somatotropin)—

Recombinant bovine somatotropin (rBST) is virtually identical to a cow's natural somatotropin, a hormone produced in its pituitary gland that stimulates milk production. Treatment with rBST can increase a cow's milk production by 10 percent to 15 percent.

Bt (Bacillus thuringiensis)—

One of the most common microorganisms used in biologically-based pesticides is the Bacillus thuringiensis or Bt bacterium. Several of the proteins produced by the Bt, principally in the coating the bacteria forms around itself, are lethal to individual species of insects. By using Bt in pesticide formulations, target insects can be controlled using an environmentally benign, biologically-based agent. Bt-based insecticides have been widely used by home gardeners for many years as well as on farms.

Bulimia Nervosa—

An eating disorder characterized by rapid consumption of a large amount of food in a short period of time, with a sense of lack of control during the episode and self-evaluation unduly influenced by body weight and shape. There are two forms of the condition, purging and non-purging. The first type regularly engages in purging through self-induced vomiting or the excessive use of laxatives or diuretics. Alternatively, the non-purging type controls weight through strict dieting, fasting or excessive exercise.

butylated hydroxyanisole (BHA)—

A phenolic chemical compound used to preserve foods by preventing rancidity. It may also be used as a defoaming agent for yeast. BHA is found in foods high in fats and oils; also in meats, cereals, baked goods, beer, and snack foods.

butylated hydroxytoluene (BHT)—

A phenolic chemical compound used to keep food from changing flavor, odor and/or color. It is added to foods high in fats and oils and cereals.

Back to top

Cc

caffeic acid—

A type of phenol found in various fruits, vegetables and citrus fruits which has antioxidant like activities that may reduce the risk of degenerative diseases, heart disease and eye disease.

caffeine—

Caffeine is a naturally-occurring substance found in the leaves, seeds or fruits of over 63 plant species worldwide and is part of a group of compounds known as methylxanthines. The most commonly known sources of caffeine are coffee and cocoa beans, cola nuts and tea leaves. Caffeine is a pharmacologically active substance and, depending on the dose, can be a mild central nervous system stimulant. Caffeine does not accumulate in the body over the course of time and is normally excreted within several hours of consumption.

calcium—

A mineral that builds bones and strengthens bones, helps in muscle contraction and heartbeat, assists with nerve functions and blood clotting. Teens 18 years and younger should strive to consume about 1,300 milligrams per day. Individuals 50 years and older need about 1,200 milligrams per day. Everyone else should strive for about 1,000 milligrams per day. Milk and other diary foods such as yogurt and most cheeses are the best sources of calcium. In addition, dark green leafy vegetables, fish with edible bones, and calcium fortified foods supply significant amounts.

calorie—

A calorie is the amount of energy required to raise the temperature of one milliliter (ml) of water at a standard initial temperature by one degree centigrade (1°C).

carbohydrate—

Carbohydrates are organic compounds that consist of carbon, hydrogen and oxygen. They vary from simple sugars containing from three to seven carbon atoms to very complex polymers. Only the hexoses (sugars with six carbon atoms) and pentoses (sugars with five carbon atoms) and their polymers play important roles in nutrition. Carbohydrates in food provide 4 calories per gram.

Plants manufacture and store carbohydrates as their chief source of energy. The glucose synthesized in the leaves of plants is used as the basis for more complex forms of carbohydrates. Classification of carbohydrates relates to their structural core of simple sugars, saccharides. Principal monosaccharides that occur in food are glucose and fructose. Three common disaccharides are sucrose, maltose and lactose. Polysaccharides of interest in nutrition include starch, dextrin, glycogen and cellulose.

carcinogens, natural and synthetic—

The basic mechanism involved in the entire process of carcinogenisis—from exposure to the organism to expression of tumors—are qualitatively similar, if not identical, for the synthetic and naturally occurring carcinogens. Consequently, both naturally occurring and synthetic chemicals can be evaluated by the same epidemiologic or experimental methods and procedures.

caries—

see <u>dental caries</u>

Center for Disease Control and Prevention (CDC)—

The CDC, composed of 11 Centers, Institutes and Offices, aims to promote health and quality of life by preventing and controlling disease, injury and disability.

carrageenan—

A compound extracted from Irish moss (a type of seaweed) that is used in puddings, milk shakes and ice cream to stabilize and keep color and flavor even.

catechins—

A type of flavonoid found in tea which provides the health benefits of neutralizing free radicals and possibly reducing the risk of cancer.

cholesterol (dietary)—

Cholesterol is not a fat, but rather a fat-like substance classified as a lipid. Cholesterol is vital to life and is found in all cell membranes. It is necessary for the production of bile acids and steroid hormones. Dietary cholesterol is found only in animal foods. Abundant in organ meats and egg yolks, cholesterol is also contained in meats and poultry. Vegetable oils and shortenings are cholesterol-free.

cholesterol (serum, or blood)—

High blood cholesterol is a risk factor in the development of coronary heart disease. Most of the cholesterol that is found in the blood is manufactured by the body, in the liver, at a rate of about 800 to 1,500 milligrams a day. By comparison, the average American consumes 300 to 450 milligrams daily in foods.

cholesterol (different types)—

Blood cholesterol is divided into three separate classes of lipoproteins: very-low density lipoprotein (VLDL); low-density lipoprotein (LDL), which contains most of the cholesterol found in the blood; and high-density lipoprotein (HDL).

LDL seems to be the culprit in coronary heart disease and is popularly known as the "bad cholesterol." By contrast, HDL is increasingly considered desirable and known as the "good cholesterol."

chromosome—

Thread-like components in the cell that contain DNA. They make proteins. Genes are carried on the chromosomes.

clinical trials—

Clinical trials undertake experimental study of human subjects. Trials may attempt to determine whether the finds of basic research are applicable to humans, or to confirm the results of epidemiological research. Studies may be small, with a limited number of participants, or they may be large intervention trials that seek to discover the outcome of treatments on entire populations. The "gold standard" clinical trials are double-blind, placebo-controlled studies which employ random assignment of subjects to experimental and control groups unknown to the subject or the researcher.

confounding variable or confounding factor—

A "hidden" variable that may cause an association which the researcher attributes to other variables.

collagen hydrolysate—

A functional component of gelatin which may help improve some symptoms associated with osteoarthritis.

conjugated lenoleic acid (CLA)—

A type of fatty acid found in cheeses and some meat products which may provide the health benefits of improving body composition and decreasing the risk of certain cancers.

Continuing Survey of Food Intake of Individuals (CSFII)—

A part of the National Nutrition Monitoring System which was the first nationwide dietary intake survey designed to be conducted annually. The survey is conducted by the USDA.

control group—

The group of subjects in a study to whom a comparison is made in order to determine whether an observation or treatment has an effect. In an experimental study it is the group that does not receive a treatment. Subjects are as similar as possible to those in the test or treatment group.

controlled experiment—

In this type of research, study subjects (whether animal or human) are selected according to relevant characteristics, and then randomly assigned to either an experimental group, or a control group. Random assignment ensures that factors known as variables, which may affect the outcome of the study, are distributed equally among the groups and therefore could not lead to differences in the effect of the treatment under study. The experimental group is then given a treatment (sometimes called an intervention), and the results are compared to the control group, which does not receive treatment. A placebo, or false treatment, may be administered to the control group. With all other variables controlled, differences between the experimental and control groups may be attributed to the treatment under study.

correlation—

An association, or when one phenomenon is found to be accompanied by another. A correlation does not prove cause and effect. Correlation may also be defined statistically.

crop residues—

Plant materials remaining from the former crop that are left on the soil surface after planting form crop residues. Crop residues reduce soil erosion, air and surface water pollution, conserve soil moisture, and improve the soil by adding organic matter.

crustacean—

Any of the various aquatic arthropods, including lobsters, crabs, shrimps and barnacles. Characteristically have segmented bodies, chitinous exoskeletons and paired, jointed limbs.

cultural controls—

An integrated pest management method which includes annual crop rotation to discourage pests and weed production.

cyclamate—

A sweetener which is 30 times sweeter than sucrose, calorie free and heat stable and works synergistically with other sweeteners. It is approved for table-top use in Canada and more than 50 countries in Europe, Asia, South America and Africa. Since 1970, however, the use of cyclamate has been banned in the United States on the basis of a study that suggested that cyclamates may be related to the development of bladder tumors in rats. Although 75 subsequent studies have failed to show that cyclamate is carcinogenic, the sweetener has yet to be reapproved for use in the United States.

Back to top

Dd

dental caries—

Popularly known as cavities, dental caries occur when bacteria in the mouth feed on fermentable carbohydrates and produce acids that dissolve tooth enamel. Various conditions affect this process, such as heredity and the composition and flow of saliva. Any fermentable carbohydrate (starches and sugars) can serve as food for cavity-causing bacteria. The amount of carbohydrate is not as important as how often these foods are eaten and how long they stay in the mouth. Widespread use of fluoride in water supplies and oral health products is credited with the dramatic decline in dental caries among children and adults alike over the past 20 years. Also, see "fluoride."

diabetes—

Diabetes is the name for a group of medical disorders characterized by high blood sugar levels. Normally when people eat, food is digested and much of it is converted to glucose—a simple sugar—which the body uses for energy.

The blood carries the glucose to cells where it is absorbed with the help of the hormone insulin. For those with diabetes, however, the body does not make enough insulin, or cannot properly use the insulin it does make. Without insulin, glucose accumulates in the blood rather than moving into the cells. High blood sugar levels result.

diallyl sulfide—

A type of sulfide/thoil found in onions, garlic, olives, leeks and scallions which may provide the health benefits of lowering LDL cholesterol and of maintaining a healthy immune system.

Dietary Guidelines for Americans—

Issued by the United States Department of Agriculture and the Department of Health and Human Services (USDA/DHHS) every five years, the Dietary Guidelines are based on scientific consensus and form the cornerstone of federal nutrition policy. The fifth edition, issued in 2000, contains ten guidelines. Its message, built around three actions "Aim, Build and Choose," strives to motivate Americans with the following advice: 1) Aim for Fitness 2) Build a Healthy Base and 3) Choose sensibly. This revised set of guidelines is the first to recommend daily physical activity and the first to include a guideline specific to food safety.

DNA—

Also known as Deoxyribonucleic acid. This is the molecule that carries the genetic information for most living systems. The DNA molecule consists of four bases (adenine, cytosine, guanine and thymine) and a sugar-phosphate backbone, arranged in two connected strands to form its characteristic double-helix.

double-blind placebo-controlled study—

Considered the "gold standard" of clinical research studies, the double-blind placebo-controlled study provides dependable findings that are free of bias introduced by either the subject or the researcher. In this type of study, neither the subject nor the researcher conducting the study know whether the test substance or a placebo has been administered. For the results to be valid and to ensure that the subject cannot violate the "blindness," the placebo and the test substance must be virtually identical (i.e., look, smell and taste similar). The "blindness" of the study is crucial. It eliminates the possibility that a participant's personal beliefs will undermine the study's validity. It also prevents the researcher's expectations from influencing the test results.

Back to top

Ee

E. coli: O157:H7—

The bacteria Escherichia coli: O157:H7 is a type of E. coli associated with foodborne illness. Healthy cattle and humans can carry the bacteria. It can be transferred from animal to animal and animal to human, and from animal to human on food. Transmission from person to person through close contact is a potential problem, especially among young children in daycare.

eating disorders—

Eating disorders may be classified as anorexia, bulimia, compulsive overeating, binge eating, or any combination of these. Each is based on specific diagnostic criteria.

ecologist—

An individual who studies the interrelationships between organisms and their environment.

ellagic acid—

A natural-cancer fighting agent found in strawberries.

endocrine disruption—

Not considered as an adverse endpoint per se but as a step or mechanism that could lead to toxic outcomes, such as cancer or adverse reproductive effects.

enriched foods—

Enriched foods are those that nutrients have been added to replace the nutrients which were lost during food processing. For example, B vitamins are lost in processing wheat to white flour and these are then added back to the flour.

Environmental Protection Agency (EPA)—

The EPA's mission is to protect human health and safeguard the natural environment—air, water and land—upon which life depends. Through regulation, EPA tries to ensure the human population and the environment are protected from environmental risks and exposures.

epidemiology—

The study of distribution and determinants of diseases or other health outcomes in human populations. It seeks to expose potential associations between aspects of health (such as cancer, heart disease, etc.) and diet, lifestyle, habits or other factors within populations. Epidemiological studies may suggest relationships between two factors, but do not provide the basis for conclusions about cause and effect. Possible associations inferred from epidemiological research can turn out to be coincidental.

epinephrine—

An adrenal hormone that stimulates autonomic nerve reaction. It is used in the treatment of anaphylaxis to open airways and blood vessels.

experimental group—

The group of subjects in an experimental study which receives a treatment.

Back to top

Ff

fat replacers—

Fat replacers are developed to duplicate the taste and texture of fat, but contain fewer calories per gram than fat. Fat replacers generally fall into three categories: carbohydrate-, protein- or fat-based. The ingredients that are used to replace fat depend on how the food product will be eaten or prepared. For example, not all fat replacer ingredients are heat stable. Thus, the fat replacer that worked well in a salad dressing may not work well in a muffin mix.

fats (dietary fats)—

Fats are referred to in the plural because there is no one type of fat. Fats are composed of the same three elements as carbohydrates—carbon, hydrogen and oxygen, However, fats have relatively more carbon and hydrogen and less oxygen, thus supplying a higher fuel value of nine calories per gram (versus four calories per gram from carbohydrates and protein).

One molecule of fat can be broken down into three molecules of fatty acids and one molecule of glycerol. Thus, fats are known chemically as triglycerides.

Fats are a vital nutrient in a healthy diet. Fats supply essential fatty acids, such as linoleic acid, which is especially important to childhood growth. Fat helps maintain healthy skin, regulate cholesterol metabolism and is a precursor of prostaglandins, hormone-like substances that regulate some body processes. Dietary fat is needed to carry fat-soluble vitamins A, D, E and K and to aid in their absorption from the intestine.

fatty acid—

Fatty acids are generally classified as saturated, monounsaturated or polyunsaturated. These terms refer to the number of hydrogen atoms attached to the carbon atoms of the fat molecule. In general, fats that contain a majority of saturated fatty acids are solid at room temperature, although some solid vegetable shortenings are up to 75 percent unsaturated. Fats containing mostly unsaturated fatty acids are usually liquid at room temperature and are called oils. Also, see "fats", or "hydrogenation."

fertilizer—

Any organic or inorganic material, either natural or synthetic, used to supply elements (such as nitrogen, phosphate and potash) essential for plant growth. If used in excess or attached to eroding soil, fertilizers can become a source of water pollution.

ferulic acid—

A type of phenol found in various fruits and vegetables and citrus fruits which has antioxidant like activities that may reduce the risk of degenerative diseases, heart disease and eye disease.

fiber—

Dietary fiber generally refers to parts of fruits, vegetables, grains, nuts and legumes that can't be digested by humans. Meats and dairy products do not contain fiber. Studies indicate that high-fiber diets can reduce the risks of heart disease and certain types of cancer. There are two basic types of fiber—insoluble and soluble. Soluble fiber in cereals, oatmeal, beans and other foods has been found to lower blood cholesterol. Insoluble fiber in cauliflower, cabbage and other vegetables and fruits helps move foods through the stomach and intestine, thereby decreasing the risk of cancers of the colon and rectum.

5 A Day—

Refers to the dietary recommendation to consume five servings of fruits and vegetables every day. The tagline, 5 A Day, became a promotional message in campaigns to increase fruits and vegetable consumption.

flavanones—

A type of flavonoid found in citrus fruits which provides the health benefits of neutralizing free radicals and possibly reducing the risk of cancer.

flavones—

A type of flavonoid found in various fruits and vegetables which provides the health benefits of neutralizing free radicals and possibly reducing the risk of cancer.

fluoride—

Fluoride is a natural component of minerals in rocks and soils. Widespread use of fluoride in water supplies and oral health products is credited with the dramatic decline in dental caries among children and adults alike. All water contains fluoride, but it is sometimes necessary to add it to some public supplies to attain the optimal amount for dental health. Fluoride makes tooth enamel stronger and more resistant to decay. It also prevents the growth of harmful bacteria and interferes with converting fermentable carbohydrates to acids in the mouth.

folic acid—

Folic acid, folate, folacin, all form a group of compounds functionally involved in amino acid metabolism and nucleic acid synthesis. Good dietary sources of folate include leafy, dark green vegetables, legumes, citrus fruits and juices, peanuts, whole grains and fortified breakfast cereals.

Recent studies show, if all women of childbearing age consumed sufficient folic acid (either through diet or supplements), 50 to 70 percent of birth defects of the brain and spinal cord could be prevented, according to the U.S. Centers for Disease Control and Prevention (CDC.) Folic acid is critical from conception through the first four to six weeks of pregnancy when the neural tube is formed. This means adequate diet or supplement use should begin before pregnancy occurs.

Recent research findings also show low blood folate levels can be associated with elevated plasma homocysteine and increased risk of coronary heart disease.

Food and Drug Administration (FDA)—

The Food and Drug Administration is part of the Public Health Service of the U.S. Department of Health and Human Services. It is the regulatory agency responsible for ensuring the safety and wholesomeness of all foods sold in interstate commerce except meat, poultry and eggs (which are under the jurisdiction of the U.S. Department of Agriculture). FDA develops standards for the composition, quality, nutrition, safety and labeling of foods including food and color additives. It conducts research to improve detection and prevention of contamination. It collects and interprets data on nutrition, food additives and pesticide residues. The agency also inspects food plants, imported food products and feed mills that make feeds containing medications or nutritional supplements that are destined for human consumption. And it regulates radiation-emitting products such as microwave ovens. FDA also enforces pesticide tolerances established by the Environmental Protection Agency for all domestically produced and imported foods, except for foods under USDA jurisdiction.

Food Guide Pyramid—

The Food Guide Pyramid is a graphic design used to communicate the recommended daily food choices contained in the Dietary Guidelines for Americans. The information provided was developed and promoted by the U.S. Department of Agriculture and the U.S. Department of Health and Human Services.

food idiosyncrasy—

Non-allergic reaction to food or food component that occurs through unknown mechanisms.

food intolerance—

A general term for any adverse reaction to a food or food component that does not involve the body's immune system.

food irradiation—

The exposure of food to sufficient radiant energy (gamma rays, x-rays and electron beams) to destroy microorganisms and insects. Irradiation is used in food production and processing to promote food safety.

food preservatives—

All preservatives prevent spoilage either by slowing the growth of organisms that live on food or by protecting the food from oxygen. Antimicrobials are preservatives that protect food by slowing the growth of bacteria, molds and yeasts. Antioxidants are preservatives that protect by preventing food molecules from combining with oxygen (air).

Food Quality Protection Act (FQPA)—

A law (enacted in August 1996) which significantly amended the Federal Insecticide, Fungicide and Rodenticide Act (FIFRA) and the Federal Food, Drug and Cosmetic Act (FFDCA) and thus provided increased protection for infants and children from pesticide risk. The new safety standard resulting from FQPA is a "reasonable certainty of no harm" standard for aggregate exposure using dietary residues and all other reliable exposure information.

food safety—

Food safety is a relative and not absolute matter. Relative food safety can be defined as the practical, certainty that injury or damage will not result from food or ingredient used in reasonable and customary manner and quantity.

foodborne disease—

Disease, usually gastrointestinal, caused by organisms or their toxins carried in ingested food. Also commonly known as "food poisoning."

fortified foods—

Fortified foods have nutrients added to them that were not present originally. For example, milk is fortified with vitamin D, which helps your body absorb calcium and phosphorus found naturally in milk.

Free radical—

Highly reactive substances that result from exposure to oxygen, background radiation, and other environmental factors. These free radicals cause cellular damage in the body. The damage may be repaired by antioxidants.

fructo-oliogosaccharides (FSO)—

A type of prebiotic/probiotic found in Jerusalem artichokes, shallots and onion powder which may improve gastrointestinal health.

fructose—

Fructose is a monosaccharide found naturally in fruits, as an added sugar in a crystalline form and as a component of high-fructose corn syrup (HFCS).

fruit—

Fruit is the usually edible reproductive body of a seed plant, especially one having a sweet pulp associated with the seed.

functional component—

Those components in food that provide special health benefits. The abilities of these functional components may reduce cancer risk, aid digestion, decrease risk of tooth decay or improve various other body functions or reduce disease risk.

functional foods—

Foods that may provide health benefits beyond basic nutrition. Examples include tomatoes with lycopene, thought to help prevent the incidence of prostate and cervical cancers; fiber in wheat bran and sulfur compounds in garlic also believed to prevent cancer.

fungicide—

A chemical that is mixed with wax and applied to fruits or vegetables to prevent mold and rot from developing.

Back to top

Gg

galactose—

A monosaccharide occurring in both levo (L) and dextro (D) forms as a constituent of plant and animal oligosaccharides (lactose and raffinose) and polysaccharides (agar and pectin). Galactose is the sugar derived from digesting lactose ("milk sugar").

gallbladder disease—

There are several different forms of gallbladder disease: 1) *Gallstones without symptoms.* About 20% of women and 8% of men will develop gallstones. In most of these cases, gallstones do not produce symptoms and thus usually do not require treatment. 2) *Biliary colic.* This condition occurs when a gallstone intermittently blocks the duct that drains the gallbladder (cystic duct). Biliary colic usually causes severe, steady pain that lasts from 15 to 60 minutes to up to 6 hours. 3) *Inflammation of the gallbladder (acute cholecystitis).* This condition occurs when a gallstone becomes stuck in the cystic duct, causing severe abdominal pain that lasts longer then 6 hours. It is the most common complication of gallstone disease. 4) *Chronic cholecystitis.* This condition develops when there is long term (chronic) inflammation of the gallbladder. The wall of the gallbladder may be thickened and rigid. 5) *Common bile duct stones (choledocholithiasis).* This condition occurs when a gallstone passes through the cystic duct into the common bile duct. About 8 to 15% of people who have gallstones also have common bile duct stones. Most people who have common bile duct stones do not have symptoms. However, people who do have symptoms may develop life-threatening complications, such as infection and inflammation of the bile duct or pancreas.

gastronomy—

The study and appreciation of good food and good eating, and a culture's culinary customs, style and lore. Any interest or study of culinary pursuits as relates essentially to the kitchen and cookery, and to the higher levels of education, training and achievement of the chef apprentice or professional chef.

gene—

A natural unit of the hereditary material, which is the physical basis for the transmission of the characteristics of living organisms from one generation to another. The basic genetic material is fundamentally the same in all living organisms; it consists of chain-like molecules of nucleic acids—deoxyribonucleic acid (DNA) in most organisms and ribonucleic acid (RNA) in certain viruses—and is usually associated in a linear arrangement that (in part) constitutes a chromosome.

generalizability—

The extent to which the results of a study are able to be applied to the general population of people that is comparable to the population studied.

genetic engineering/genetic modification/genetic enhancement—

The selective, deliberate alteration of genes (genetic material) by man. This term has a very broad meaning including the manipulation and alteration of the genetic material of an organism in such a way as to allow it to produce endogenous proteins with properties different from those of the normal, or to produce entirely different (foreign) proteins altogether. Other words applicable to the same process are gene splicing, gene manipulation, or recombinant DNA technology.

genome—

The total hereditary material of a cell, containing the entire chromosomal set found in each nucleus of a given species.

glucose—

A sugar, most commonly in the form of dextroglucose, that occurs naturally, has about half the sweetening power of regular sugar and does not crystallize easily. Glucose comes from grape juice, honey and certain vegetables, among other things.

glutamate—

Glutamate is an amino acid. It is necessary for metabolism and brain function, and is manufactured by the body. Glutamate is found in virtually every protein food we eat. In food, there is "bound" glutamate and "free" glutamate. Glutamate serves to enhance flavors in foods when it is in its free form and not bound to other amino acids in protein. Some foods have greater quantities of glutamate than others. Foods that are rich in glutamate include tomatoes, mushrooms, parmesan cheese, milk and mackerel.

glycerin—

A syrupy type of alcohol derived from sugar which is used in food flavorings to maintain desired food consistency.

glycerol—

A colorless, odorless, syrupy liquid—chemically, an alcohol—that is obtained from fats and oils and used to retain moisture and add sweetness to foods.

Good Manufacturing Practices (GMP)—

The Food and Drug Administration's (FDA's) approval mechanism for a process to manufacture a given food or food additive. It is implemented instead of specific regulations (such as those used to dictate processes in simple food manufacturing, as in beef packing), due to the newness of the technology and may later be superceded (due to further advances in the technology).

grains—

Grains are the seeds or fruits of various food plants including cereal grasses. The examples of wheat, corn, oats, barley, rye and rice provide a partial list. Grain foods include foods such as bread, cereals, rice and pasta.

GRAS (Generally Recognized as Safe)—

GRAS is the regulatory status of food ingredients not evaluated by the FDA prescribed testing procedure. It also includes common food ingredients that were already in use when the 1959 Food Additives Amendment to the Food, Drug and Cosmetic Act was enacted.

guar gum—

A substance made from the seeds of the guar plant which acts as a stabilizer in food systems. Is found as a food additive in cheese, including processed cheese, ice cream and dressings.

Back to top

Hb

HACCP (Hazard Analysis and Critical Control Points)—

The underlying approach under HACCP for preventing foodborne illness and promote quality is to identify the danger spots and try to avoid them. Instead of putting the burden on government to discover that a food safety problem exists, HACCP shifts responsibility onto the industry to ensure that the food it produces is safe. Food producers will have to prevent bacterial contamination from occurring in the first place. HACCP works by the following principles:

- Identify the likely health hazards to consumers in a given product.
- Identify the critical points in the processing where the hazards may occur.
- Establish safety measures to prevent the hazard from occurring.
- Monitor to make sure the safety measures are working.
- Establish an appropriate remedy if monitoring shows a problem.
- Establish detailed record keeping to document monitoring and remedies taken.
- Verify that the whole system is working.

health claims—

Claims that link food—or food components—in the overall diet with a lowered risk of some chronic diseases. Strictly regulated by the Food and Drug Administration, only health claims supported by scientific evidence are allowed on food labels. Since this information is optional, many foods that meet the criteria don't carry any health claim on their label.

helix—

A spiral, staircase-like structure with a repeating pattern described by two simultaneous operations (rotation and translation). It is one of the natural conformations exhibited by biological polymers.

herbicides—

Herbicides are a class of crop protection and specialty chemicals used to control weeds on farms and in forests, as well as in non-agricultural applications such as golf courses, public tracts of land and residential lawns.

high-fructose corn syrup (HFCS)—

HFCS are formulations generally containing 42 percent, 55 percent or 90 percent fructose (the remaining carbohydrate being primarily glucose) depending on the product application. HCFS are used in products such as soft drinks or cake mixes.

Human Genome Project—

This project is, in simplest terms, a sequencing of the human genome. Information from the Human Genome Project is making it possible, for example, to identify the exact gene (or genes) that influences a person's susceptibility to a disease, to develop new and better drugs, and to identify thousands of different polymorphisms. The full scope of the Human Genome Project's potential to improve human health is only beginning to be appreciated.

hybridization of crops—

The mating of two plants from different species or genetically very different members of the same species to yield hybrids possessing some of the characteristics of each parent. Those (hybrid) offspring tend to be more healthy, productive and uniform than their parents—a phenomenon known as "hybrid vigor."

hydrogenation—

Hydrogenation is the process of adding hydrogen molecules directly to an unsaturated fatty acid from sources such as vegetable oils to convert it to a semi-solid form such as margarine or shortening. Hydrogenation contributes important textural properties to food. The degree of hydrogenation influences the firmness and spreadability of margarines, flakiness of pie crust and the creaminess of puddings. Hydrogenated oils are sometimes used in place of other fats with higher proportions of saturated fatty acids such as butter or lard.

hyperactivity—

See <u>Attention Deficit Hyperactivity Disorder (ADHD)</u>.

hypertension—

Hypertension is the persistently elevated arterial blood pressure. It is the most common public health problem in developed countries. Emphasis on lifestyle modifications has given diet a prominent role for both the primary prevention and management of hypertension.

<u>Back to top</u>

Ii

immune system—

The cells and tissues which are responsible for recognizing and attacking foreign microbes and substances in the body.

immunoglobulin E—

The antibody in the immune system that reacts with allergens.

incidence—

The number of new cases of a disease during a given period of time in a defined population.

insecticide—

Insecticides are a class of crop protection and specialty chemicals used to control insects on farms and forests, as well as non-agricultural applications such as residential lawncare, golf courses and public tracts of land.

insoluble fiber—

A type of dietary fiber found in wheat bran, cauliflower, cabbage and other vegetables and fruits which helps move foods through the digestive system and thereby may decrease the risks of cancers of the colon and rectum. Insoluble fiber may also help reduce the risk of breast cancer.

integrated pest management (IPM)—

Integrated pest management is the coordinated use of pest and environmental information along with available pest control methods, including cultural, biological, genetic and chemical methods, to prevent unacceptable levels of pest damage using the most economical means, and with the least possible hazard to people, property and the environment.

intense sweeteners—

see low-calorie sweeteners

isoflavones—Daidzein, Genistein—

A type of phytoestrogen found in soybeans and soy-based foods which may reduce menopause symptoms.

Back to top

Jj

Kk

Back to top

Ll

lactobacillus—

A type of prebiotic/probiotic found in yogurt and some other dairy products which may improve gastrointestinal health.

lactose—

A sugar naturally occurring in milk, also known as "milk sugar," that is the least sweet of all natural sugars and used in baby formulas and candies.

lactose intolerance—

Lactose intolerance is an inherited inability to properly digest dairy products, due to a deficiency in the amount of the enzyme, β-galactosidase in the small intestine. This enzyme is necessary for the hydrolysis of lactose (a disaccharide) into its constituent monosaccharides, glucose and galactose. Symptoms of lactose intolerance, including abdominal cramps, flatulence and frothy diarrhea, can increase with age.

lecithin—

A by-product of the refining for soybean oil and is also found in eggs, red meats, spinach and nuts. Historically, lecithin has been used commercially in food processing as an emulsifier, instantizing agent and lubricating agent. Lecithin is a source of choline when digested; and is a critical component of the lipoproteins which transport fat and cholesterol molecules in the blood stream. Lecithin (choline) promotes synthesis of high-density lipoproteins (i.e., HDLP also know as "good" cholesterol) by the liver, when it is consumed by humans.

lignans—

A type of phytoestrogen found in flax, rye and various vegetables which may provide the health benefits of lowering LDL cholesterol, total cholesterol and triglycerides thereby protecting against heart disease and some cancers.

listeria—

Listeria monocytogenes is a Gram-positive bacterium, found in at least 37 mammalian species, as well as 17 species of birds and possibly some fish and shellfish. The bacteria can be isolated from soil, and is resistant to heat, freezing and drying.

Listeria has been associated with foods such as raw milk, soft-ripened cheeses, ice cream, raw vegetables, raw and cooked poultry, raw meat and raw and smoked fish. Unlike other pathogenic bacteria, such as salmonella, listeria can survive and grow at temperatures as low as 5°C (41°F).

Acute infection with listeria may result in flu-like symptoms including persistent fever, followed by septicemia, meningitis, encephalitis, and intrauterine or cervical infections in pregnant women. Possible gastrointestinal symptoms include nausea, vomiting and diarrhea, alone or couple with other symptoms (mentioned above).

low-calorie sweetener—

Low-calorie sweeteners are non-nutritive sweeteners, also referred to as intense sweeteners. Low-calorie sweeteners can replace nutritive sweeteners in most foods at a caloric savings of approximately 16 calories per teaspoon.

Thus, caloric reduction may be achieved when low-calorie sweetened foods and beverages are substituted for their full-calorie counterparts. Examples of low-calorie sweeteners in use in the U.S. food supply are saccharin, aspartame and acesulfame K.

lutein—

A type of carotenoid found in most green vegetables which positively contributes to maintenance of eye vision.

lycopene—

Lycopene is a carotenoid related to the better known beta-carotene. Lycopene gives tomatoes and some other fruits and vegetables their distinctive red color. Nutritionally, it functions as an antioxidant. Research shows lycopene is best absorbed by the body when consumed as tomatoes that have been heat-processed using a small amount of oil. This includes products such as tomato sauce and tomato paste. Also, see <u>functional foods</u>.

lysine—

An essential, basic amino acid obtained from many proteins by hydrolysis.

<u>Back to top</u>

Mm

Mad Cow Disease—

See <u>BSE (Bovine spongiform encephalopathy)</u>.

mast cells—

Tissue cells which when connected to immunoglobulin E antibodies release histamine or other substances causing allergic symptoms.

meta-analysis—

A quantitative technique in which the results of several individual studies are pooled to yield overall conclusions.

metabolism—

The entire set of enzyme-catalyzed transformations of organic nutrient molecules (to sustain life) in living cells. Conversion of food and water into nutrients that can be used by the body's cells, and the use of those nutrients by those cells (to sustain life, grow, etc.).

methionine—

An essential amino acid; furnishes (to organism) both labile methyl groups and sulfur necessary for normal metabolism.

methyl cellulose—

A number of gummy substances, produced through reaction between cellulose and methyls. It is found in fruit butters and jellies and serves to keep these products from separating.

microorganisms—

Simple unicellular and structurally similar representatives of the plant and animal kingdoms. With few exceptions, the unicellular organisms are invisible to the naked eye and generally have dimensions of between a fraction of a micron and 200 micron.

mono- & di-glycerides—

Emulsifying agents found in shortening, margarine, cacao products and bakery products. Usually derived from soybean fat, these food additives keep food products from separating.

MSG (monosodium glutamate)—

MSG is the sodium salt of glutamic acid. Glutamic acid, or glutamate, is one of the most common amino acids found in nature. (see <u>glutamate</u>)
In the early part of the century, MSG was extracted from seaweed and other plant sources. Today, MSG is produced in many countries around the world through a fermentation process of molasses from sugar cane or sugar beets, as well as starch and corn sugar.

morbid obesity—

This is a state of adiposity or overweight, in which body weight is 100 percent above the ideal and a body mass index of 45 or greater.

mycotoxins—

Toxins produced by fungi. More than 350 different mycotoxins are known to man. Almost all mycotoxins possess the capacity to harmfully alter the immune systems of animals. Consumption by humans and animals of certain mycotoxins (e.g., via eating infected corn, nuts, peanuts cottonseed products, etc.) can result in liver toxicity, gastrointestinal lesions, cancer and muscle necrosis.

Nn

Nationwide Food Consumption Survey (NFCS)—

A survey conducted by the USDA roughly every ten years that monitors the nutrient intake of a cross-section of the U.S. public.

National Health and Nutrition Examination Survey (NHANES)—

A series of surveys that include information from medical history, physical measurements, biochemical evaluation, physical examination and dietary intake of population groups within the United States. The NHANES is conducted by the U.S. Department of Health and Human Services approximately every five years.

natural toxins—

A naturally occurring substance (e.g., produced in some cases by disease-causing microorganisms) which is poisonous to certain other living organisms.

nematodes—

Microscopic, wormlike organisms that feed on plant roots.

neotame—

A versatile, new no-calorie sweetener composed of two elements of protein, the amino acids L-aspartic acid and L-phenylalanine, combined with two organic functional groups, a methyl ester group and a neohexyl group. It is approximately 7,000 to 13,000 times sweeter than sugar and as such captures the "essence of sweetness." with only a very small amount required for use. The chemical composition of neotame makes it stable for use in baking.

The FDA has recently approved Neotame for use in a variety of food products and as a tabletop sweetener.

neural tube defect—

In simple terms, a neural tube defect (NTD) is a malformation of the brain or spinal cord (neurological system) during embryonic development. Infants born with spina bifida, where the spinal cord is exposed, can grow to adulthood but usually suffer from paralysis or other disabilities. Babies born with anencephaly, where most or all of the brain is missing, usually die shortly after birth. These NTDs make up about 5 percent of all U.S. birth defects each year.

According to the CDC, the use of sufficient folic acid is enough to eliminate the risk of NTDs. (see <u>folic acid</u>)

nitrite—

Nitrite is a safe food additive that has been used for centuries to preserve meats, fish and poultry. It also contributes to the characteristic flavor, color and texture of processed meats such as hot dogs. Because nitrite safeguards cured meats against the most deadly foodborne bacterium of all, Clostridium (C.) botulinum, its use is supported by the public health community.
The human body generates much greater nitrite levels than are added to food. Nitrates consumed in foods such as carrots and green vegetables are converted to nitrite during digestion. Nitrite in the body is instrumental in promoting blood clotting, healing wounds and burns, and boosting immune function to kill tumor cells.

nitrogen—

A nonmetallic element that constitutes nearly four-fifths of the air by volume, occurring as a colorless, odorless, almost inert diatomic gas in various minerals and in all proteins. It is used in a wide variety of important manufacturers, including ammonia, nitric acid, TNT and fertilizers.

nitrosamines—

Nitrosamines are a digestive reaction-product of nitrite, a food additive used to preserve meats, fish and poultry. (Also see <u>nitrite</u>.)

no-till farming—

A methodology of crop production in which the farmer avoids mechanical cultivation (i.e., only one pass over the field). The plant residue remaining on the field's surface helps to control weeds and reduce soil erosion, but it also provides sites for insects to shelter and reproduce, leading to a need for increased insect control.

nutraceuticals—

One term used to describe substances in or parts of a food that may be considered to provide medical or health benefits beyond basic nutrition, including disease prevention. Research indicates this term might not appeal to consumers. Also, see "functional foods."

nutrient density—

Nutrient dense foods are those that provide substantial amounts of vitamins and minerals and relatively fewer calories. The opposite of nutrient dense is calorie dense which are foods that mainly supply calories and relatively few nutrients.

Back to top

Oo

obesity, or overweight—

Although precise definitions vary among experts, overweight has been traditionally defined as 10 percent to 20 percent above an optimal weight for height derived from statistics. Obesity is defined as body weight being 20% above normal. Some scientists argue that the amount and distribution of an individual's body fat is a significant indicator of health risk and therefore should be considered in defining overweight. Abdominal fat has been linked to more adverse health consequences than fat in the hips or thighs. Thus, calculations of waist-to-hip ratio are preferred by some health experts to help determine if an individual is overweight.

omega-3 fatty acids—DHA/EPA—

A type of fatty acid found in fish and marine oils which provide the health benefits of reduced risk of cardiovascular disease and improved mental and visual function.

organic—

Organic defines agricultural products that are grown using cultural, biological and mechanical methods prior to the use of synthetic, non-agricultural substances to control pests, improve soil quality an/or enhance processing. The USDA is currently addressing the issue of organic products, and aims to have official rules for what may be considered organic ready for the 1999 spring planting season.

Currently organic defines an agricultural process in which farmers use techniques such as crop rotation, cultivation, mulching, soil enrichment and the "encouragement" of predators and microorganisms which naturally keep pests away. The now widely accepted definition allows farmers to use natural pesticides, but nothing synthetic.

osteoporosis—

Osteoporosis is a skeletal disease in which the bones lose mass and density, the pores in bones enlarge, and the bones generally become fragile. Osteoporosis often is not diagnosed until a fracture occurs, most commonly in the spine, hip or wrist. The National Osteoporosis Foundation estimates that about 1.5 million such fractures occur each year in the United States, at an estimated annual cost of $14 billion in 1995.

Osteoporosis is four times more common in women, whose bones are naturally thinner and less dense, than in men. Women start losing bone mass and density at an earlier age, and the process is accelerated by menopause, causing osteoporosis to manifest itself between the ages of 50 and 60. Research has shown that in addition to regular exercise, calcium intake during childhood, adolescence and early-adulthood helps build a "bone bank" of calcium stores. While bone length is established by age 20, bone strength and density continue to develop through age 30.

outcomes research—

A type of research increasingly used by the health industry which provides information about how a specific procedure or treatment regimen results: the subject (clinical safety and efficacy), the subject's physical functioning and lifestyle, and economic considerations such as saving/prolonging life and avoiding costly complications.

oxidation—

The loss of electrons from a compound (or element) in a chemical reaction. When one compound is oxidized, another compound is reduced. That is, the other compound must "pick up" the electrons that the first has lost.

Back to top

Pp

palatable—

Acceptable or agreeable to taste.

pathogens—

Virus, bacterium, parasitic protozoan, or other microorganisms that cause infectious disease by invading the body of an organism know as the host. Note that infection is not synonymous with disease because infection does not always lead to injury of the host.

pectin—

A natural gelling agent found in ripe fruit. Pectin is an important ingredient in making jams and jellies. Some fruits have high pectin levels (e.g., citrus fruit, blackberries, apples and red currants) but others are low in pectin (e.g., strawberries) so lemon juice is added to strawberry jam to help the set.

pesticide—

A broad class of crop protection chemicals including four major types: insecticides used to control insects; herbicides used to control weeds; rodenticides used to control rodents; and fungicides used to control mold, mildew and fungi.

In addition consumers use pesticides in the home or yard to control termites and roaches, clean mold from shower curtains, stave off crab grass on the lawn, kill fleas and ticks on pets and disinfect swimming pools, to name just a few "specialty" pesticide uses.

pheromones—

"Sex perfume" traps used to disrupt insect reproduction cycles.

phytate—

A chemical complex (large molecule) substance that is the dominant (i.e., 60 to 80%) chemical form of phosphorous within cereal grains, oilseeds, and their by products. Monogastric animals (e.g., swine) cannot digest and utilize phosphorus within phytate, because they lack the enzyme known as phytase in their digestive system, so that phosphorus (phytate) is excreted into the environment. When phytase enzyme is present in the ration of a monogastric animal, at a high enough level, the monogastric animal is then able to digest the phytate (thereby releasing that phosphorus for absorption by the animal).

phytochemical—

Phytochemicals are substances found in edible fruits and vegetables that may be ingested by humans daily in gram quantities and that exhibit a potential for modulating the human metabolism in a manner favorable for reducing risk of cancer. (see <u>functional foods</u>)

placebo—

Sometimes casually referred to as a "sugar pill," a placebo is a "fake" treatment which seems identical to the real treatment. Placebo treatments are used to eliminate bias that may arise from the expectation that a treatment should produce an effect.

polyols—

A type of sweetener used in reduced-calorie foods. They differ from intense sweeteners in that they are considered nutritive; that is, they do contribute calories to the diet. Polyols are incompletely absorbed and metabolized, however, and consequently contribute fewer calories than sucrose. The polyols commonly used in the United States include sorbitol, mannitol, xylitol, maltitol, maltitol syrup, lactitol, erythritol, isomalt and hydrogenated starch hydrolysates. Most are approximately half as sweet as sucrose; maltitol and xylitol are about as sweet as sucrose. Polyols are found naturally in berries, apples, plums and other foods. They also are produced commercially from carbohydrates such as sucrose, glucose, and starch for use in sugar-free candies, cookies and chewing gum. Along with adding a sweet taste, polyols perform a variety of functions such as adding bulk and texture, providing a cooling effect or taste, preventing the browning that occurs during heating and retaining the moisture in foods.

post harvest waxes—

After a fruit or vegetable is picked, it continues to need moisture to stay fresh and edible. To help retain moisture, certain varieties of fresh produce are given new wax coating to replace the natural wax the fruit or vegetable loses during harvest and shipping. If a fungicide is mixed with the wax to prevent molding, retail stores must label the waxed produce.

prevalence—

The number of existing cases of a disease in a defined population at a specified time.

prion—

A prion is a rogue protein, that appears to cause Bovine spongiform encephalopathy (BSE).

proanthocyanidins—

A type of tannin found in cranberries, cranberry products, cocoa and chocolate which may provide the health benefits of improving urinary tract health and of reducing the risk of cardiovascular disease.

prospective study—

Epidemiological research that follows a group of people over a period of time to observe the potential effects of diet, behavior and other factors on health or the incidence of disease. In general, this is considered a more valid research design than retrospective research.

protein—

Chemically, a protein is a complex nitrogenous compound made up of amino acids in peptide linkages. Dietary proteins are involved in the synthesis of tissue protein and other special metabolic functions. In anabolic processes they furnish the amino acids required to build and maintain body tissues. As an energy source, proteins are equivalent to carbohydrates in providing 4 calories per gram. Proteins perform a major structural role in all body tissues and in the formation of enzymes, hormones and various body fluids and secretions. Proteins participate in the transport of some lipids, vitamins and minerals and help maintain the body's homeostasis.

Back to top

Qq

Back to top

Rr

randomization, or random assignment—

A process of assigning subjects to experimental or control groups in which the subjects have an equal chance of being assigned to each group. Randomization is used to control for known, unknown and difficult-to-control-for variables.

random sample—

A random sample is a procedure to select subjects for a study in which all individuals in a population being studied have an equal chance of being selected. using a random sample allows the results of the study to be generalized to the entire population.

The term random also applies to assignments within controlled studies, or the division of subjects into groups. Random assignment ensures that all subjects have an equal chance of being in the experimental and control groups, and increases the probability that any unidentified variable will systematically occur in both groups with the same frequency. Randomization is crucial to control for variables that researchers may not be aware of or cannot adequately control, but which could affect the outcome of an experimental study.

random sampling—

A method by which subjects are selected to participate in a study in which all individuals in a population have and equal chance of being chosen. This helps to ensure the generalizability of the study results.

rapid assays—

These diagnostic tests use emerging technology to identify and remove impurities from foods before they reach the consumer. There are two major types of rapid assays.

Antibody-based assays link a "familiar" characteristic on a pathogen's surface (the antigen) to a substance known as an antibody. When this connection is made, the test registers "success." Similarly, nucleic acid-based assays use the unique genetic materials of the cells to detect a pathogen.

recombinant DNA (rDNA)—

The DNA formed by combining segments of DNA from different organisms.

reliability—

Whether a test or instrument used to collect data, such as a questionnaire, gives the same results if repeated on the same person several times. A reliable test gives reproducible results.

rennet—

An enzyme used to make cheese. Rennet is extracted from the lining of calves' stomachs. New technologies have enabled the removal of the specific gene that produces rennet and have reproduced it in bacteria. This allows the production of rennet through a fermentation process, eliminating the need for extracts from calves' stomachs.

research design—

How a study is set up to collect information, or data. For valid results, the design must be appropriate to answer the question or hypothesis being studied.

residual confounding—

The effect that remains after one has attempted to statistically control for variables that cannot be measured perfectly. A particularly important concept in epidemiological studies because knowledge of human biology is still developing. Unknown variables could exist that could significantly change conclusions made on the basis of epidemiological research.

retrospective study—

Research that relies on recall of past data, or on previously recorded information. Often this type of research is considered to have limitations, because the number of variables that cannot be controlled, and because memory is not infallible.

risk—

A term encompassing a variety of measures of the probability of an outcome. It's usually used in reference to unfavorable outcomes such as illness or death. Be certain to distinguish between absolute and relative risk.

risk factor—

A risk factor is anything statistically shown to have a relationship with the incidence of a disease, however it does not necessarily infer cause and effect.

RNA—

Also known as ribonucleic acid. RNA is a molecule similar to DNA that functions primarily to decode the instructions carried by genes for protein synthesis.

Back to top

Ss

saccharin—

Saccharin, the oldest of the non-nutritive sweeteners, is currently produced from purified, manufactured methyl anthranilate, a substance occurring naturally in grapes. It is 300 times sweeter than sucrose, heat stable and does not promote dental caries. Saccharin has a long shelf life, but a slightly bitter aftertaste. It is not metabolized in the human digestive system, is excreted rapidly in the urine and does not accumulate in body.

salmonella—

Salmonella is a Gram-negative bacterium, occurring in many animals, especially poultry and swine. In the environment, salmonella can be found in water, soil, insects, factory and kitchen surfaces, animal fecal matter, and raw meats, poultry (including eggs) and seafood.
Acute symptoms of the illness caused by the Salmonella species include nausea, vomiting, diarrhea, abdominal cramps, headache and fever.

saponins—

The functional component of soybeans, soy foods and soy protein-containing food which may lower LDL cholesterol and may contain anti-cancer enzymes.

saturated fat—

Saturated fats are those in which all carbons contain a hydrogen, and therefore, no double bonds exist. In general, fats that contain a majority of saturated fatty acids are solid at room temperature, although some solid vegetable shortenings are up to 75 percent unsaturated. Some common fatty acids in foods include palmitic, stearic and myristic acids. Saturated fatty acids are more stable than unsaturated fatty acids because of their chemical structure. Stability is important to prevent rancidity and off flavors and odors.

selective breeding—

This process allows for the transfer of only one or a few desirable genes, thereby permitting scientists to develop crops with specific beneficial traits and those without undesirable traits. Current technology allows scientists to alter one plant characteristic at a time, thereby not spending years trying to develop the tastiest and hardiest plants.

self fixer—

The innate ability of legumes like soybeans to "fix" nitrogen, which means to use the natural nitrogen in the soil and air. These natural nitrogen fixers replenish the nitrogen supply in the soil from which they were harvested. Breeders desire to develop other crops that can "fix" their own nitrogen which would thereby decrease farmers' use of synthetic fertilizers while maintaining bountiful yields.

sodium nitrite—

A salt used in smoked or cured fish and in meat-curing preparation. It acts as a preservative and color fixative. Can combine with chemicals in the stomach to form nitrosamine, a carcinogenic substance.

soluble fiber—

A type of dietary fiber found in psyllium, cereals, oatmeal, apples, citrus fruits, beans and other foods which increases the viscosity in the gut and acts to reduce high blood cholesterol levels which decreases the risk of cardiovascular disease.

soy protein—

The protein found in soybeans and soy-based foods which when consumed at the level of 25 grams per day may reduce the risk of heart disease.

spina bifida—

Spina bifida is a birth defect in which the infant is born with the spinal cord exposed. These children can grow to adulthood although they often suffer from paralysis and other disabilities. Also, see "neural tube defects (NTDs)."

stanol/sterol esters—

A functional component found in wood oils, corn, soy and wheat which may reduce the risk of coronary heart disease by lowering blood cholesterol levels.

staple crops—

Those crops which are most common in people's diets are considered staple crops. Staple crops of greatest importance include rice, wheat and maize (corn). These three crops provide 60 percent of the world's food energy intake. And rice feeds almost half of humanity. Typically, staple crops are well adapted to the conditions in their source areas. For example, they may be tolerant of drought, pests or soils low in nutrients.

statistical power—

A mathematical quantity that indicates the probability a study has of obtaining a statistically significant effect. A high power of 80 percent, or 0.8, indicates that the study—if conducted repeatedly—would produce a statistically significant effect 80 percent of the time. On the other hand, a power of only 0.1 means there would be a 90 percent chance that the research missed the effect—if one exists at all.

statistical significance—

The probability of obtaining an effect or association in a study sample as or more extreme that the one observed if there was actually no effect in the population. Based on the hypothesis that if there truly is no effect, the results of a study are unlikely to have occurred. A P value of less than five percent (P<0.05) means the result would occur less than five percent of the time if there were no effect, and is generally considered evidence of a true treatment effect or a true relationship.

stearate—

A saturated fatty acid containing eighteen carbon atoms in its molecular "backbone" that is essentially neutral in effect on coronary heart disease in humans (i.e., doesn't appreciably increase low-density lipoproteins in the bloodstream). Because of the heart disease neutrality and resistance to oxidation/breakdown, stearate-containing oils are an excellent cooking oil choice.

sucralose—

Sucralose is the only low-calorie sweetener that is made from sugar. It is approximately 600-times sweeter and does not contain calories. Sucralose is highly stable under a wide variety of processing conditions. Thus, it can be used virtually anywhere sugar can, including cooking and baking, without losing any of its sugar-like sweetness.

Currently, sucralose is approved in over 25 countries around the world for use in food and beverages. In the US, the FDA has been petitioned to approve the use of sucralose in 15 different food and beverage categories.

sucrose—

Sucrose, a type of sugar, is a diglyceride composed of glucose and fructose. Also, see "carbohydrates."

sugar—

Although the consumer is confronted by a wide variety of sugars—sucrose, raw sugar, turbinado sugar, brown sugar, honey, corn syrup—there is no significant difference in the nutritional content or energy each provides, and therefore no advantage of one nutritionally over another. There also is no evidence that the body can distinguish between naturally occurring or added sugars in food products.

sugar alcohols—

Ingredients used to add sweet flavors to food. Those often used instead of sugars include sorbitol, mamitol, and xylitol. Many fruits and vegetables contain sugar alcohols naturally. They're also found in some sugarless gum, hard candies, jams and jellies. Besides adding sweetness, sugar alcohols also add texture, help foods stay moist, prevent browning when food is heated and give a cooling effect to the taste of food. They supply four calories per gram, but are absorbed slowly and incompletely and thus require little or no insulin for metabolism. They are not cavity-producing because they are not metabolized by bacteria that produce cavities.

sulfites—

Sulfiting agents are sometimes used to preserve the color of foods such as dried fruits and vegetable, and to inhibit the growth of microorganisms in fermented foods such as wine. Sulfites are safe for most people. A small segment of the population, however, has been found to develop shortness of breath or fatal shock shortly after exposure to these preservatives. Sulfites can provoke severe asthma attacks in sulfite-sensitive asthmatics. For that reason, in 1986 the FDA banned the use of sulfites on fresh fruits and vegetables (except potatoes) intended to be sold or served raw to consumers. Sulfites added to all packaged and processed foods must be listed on the product label.

sulphoraphane—

A functional component of cruciferous vegetables (e.g., broccoli, kale, horseradish) which provides the health benefits of neutralizing free radicals and possibly reducing the risk of cancer.

synergistic effect—

The effect achieved by the combination of two or more substances or organisms which neither alone could accomplish.

Back to top

Tt

thermal effect of food—

The increase in energy expenditure associated with the processes of digestion, absorption and metabolism of food; represents approximately 10% of a person's total energy expenditure and includes facultative thermogenesis and obligatory thermogenesis; often called diet-induced thermogenesis (DIT).

toxicologist—

A scientist who studies the nature, effects and detection of poisons and the treatment of poisoning.

toxicology—

The scientific study of the chemistry effects and treatment of poisonous substances.

traditional crop breeding—

For traditional crop breeding, breeders mix thousands of genes in order to transfer the protein products to enhance one or a few genetic traits. Therefore, the odds of something undesirable being transferred unintentionally are far greater in traditional breeding than in biotechnology.

trans fats—

Trans fats occur naturally in beef, butter, milk and lamb fats and in commercially prepared, partially hydrogenated margarines and solid cooking fats. The main sources of trans fats in the American diet today are margarine, shortening, commercial frying fats and high-fat baked goods.
Partially hydrogenated vegetable oils were developed in part to help displace highly saturated animal and vegetable fats used in frying, baking and spreads. However, trans fats, like saturated fats, raise blood LDL cholesterol levels (the so-called "bad" cholesterol). High consumption of trans fats may also reduce the HDL or "good" cholesterol levels.

Type I diabetes—

Insulin dependent (Type I) diabetes is less common than Type II. This disease occurs when the pancreas can't make insulin, or at least not enough.

Often this form of diabetes begins in childhood or the young adult years, but people of any age can get it. Insulin shots are required daily.

Type II diabetes—

Non-insulin dependent (Type II) diabetes is the more common type of diabetes and people of African-American, Hispanic and Native American decent are at higher risk of this disease. The disease develops slowly and usually becomes evident after age 40. Being overweight is a common risk factor. Often it can be controlled through diet, weight control and exercise.

Back to top

Uu

umami—

In addition to the four main taste components (sweet, sour, salty and bitter), there is the additional taste characteristic called "umami" or savory. One of the food components responsible for the umami flavor in foods is glutamate, an amino acid. Also, see "glutamate" and "MSG."

U.S. Department of Agriculture (USDA)—

The United States Department of Agriculture comprises of many agencies charged with different tasks related to agriculture and our food supply. Among these is ensuring a safe, affordable, nutritious and accessible food supply. The USDA also enhances the quality of life for the American population by supporting production of agricultural products; caring for agricultural, forest and range lands; supporting sound development of our rural communities; providing economic opportunities for farm and rural residents; expanding global markets for agricultural and forest products and services; and working to reduce hunger in America and throughout the world.

Back to top

Vv

validity—

The extent to which a study or study instrument measures what it is intended to measure. Refers to accuracy or truthfulness in regard to a study's conclusion.

variable—

Any characteristic that may vary in study subjects, such as gender, age, body weight, diet, behavior, attitude or other attribute. In an experiment, the treatment is called the independent variable; it is the factor being investigated. The variable that is influenced by the treatment is the dependent variable; it may change as a result of the effect of the independent variable.

vegetarian—

According to the Vegetarian Resource Group, less than 1 percent of Americans are true vegetarians. Such people never eat meat, fish or poultry, although they may eat foods derived from animals such as dairy products and eggs (lacto-ovo vegetarians). There are even fewer vegans, strict vegetarians who avoid all animal-derived foods—even honey.

virus—

A simple, noncellular particle (entity) that can reproduce only inside living cells (of other organisms). The simple structure of viruses is their most important characteristic. Most viruses consist only of a genetic material—either DNA or RNA—and a protein coating. Viruses are "alive" in that they can reproduce themselves, but they have none of the other characteristics of living organisms. Viruses cause a large variety of significant diseases in plants and animals, including humans.

vitamins—

Vitamins are organic compounds that are nutritionally essential in small amounts to control metabolic processes and cannot be synthesized by the body. Vitamins are usually classified by their solubility, which to some degree determines their stability; occurrence in foodstuffs; distribution in body fluids, and tissue storage capacity.

Each of the fat-soluble vitamins A, D, E and K has a distinct and separate physiologic role. Several have antioxidant properties to depress the effects of metabolic byproducts called free radicals, which are thought to cause degenerative changes related to aging.

Most of the water-soluble vitamins are components of essential enzyme systems. Many are involved in the reactions supporting energy metabolism. These vitamins are not normally stored in the body in appreciable amounts and are normally excreted in the urine. Thus, a daily supply is desirable to avoid depletion and interruption of normal physiologic functions.

Back to top

Ww

water—

Although deficiencies of energy or nutrients can be sustained for months or even years, a person can survive only a few days without water. Experts rank water second only to oxygen as essential for life. In addition to offering true refreshment for the thirsty, water plays a vital role in all bodily processes. It supplies the medium in which various chemical changes of the body occur, aiding in digestion, absorption, circulation and lubrication of body joints. For example, as a major component of blood, water helps deliver nutrients to body cells and removes waste to the kidneys for excretion.

whole grains—

The whole kernel of grain which includes the bran (outer shell), germ (nutrient rich core) and endosperm (starchy portion). The health benefit provided by whole grains is the reduced risk of cardiovascular disease which results from the combination of fiber, vitamins, minerals and phytochemicals found in whole grains.

WIC—

Special Supplemental Nutrition Program for Women, Infants, and Children. Established in 1972, the WIC program provides food and nutrition education to improve the nutritional status of medically high-risk pregnant and lactating women and children up to 5 years of age from low-income families. The program is administered by the U.S. Department of Agriculture.

Back to top

Xx

xenobiotics—

Synthetic chemicals believed to be resistant to environmental degradation. A branch of biotechnology called bioremediation is seeking to develop biological methods to degrade such compounds.

Back to top

Yy

Back to top

Zz

zeaxanthin—

A type of carotenoid found in eggs, citrus fruits and corn which positively contributes to the maintenance of eye vision.

◆   ◆   ◆

Phytonutrient News Update

(Note: Xanthones are not listed on the latest 2005 update (at the time this book went to press) of IFIC's Glossary of Food-Related Terms. Xanthones refer to a broad spectrum of a new class of phytonutrients. Xanthones are found in certain fruits, such as Mangosteen. There are several classes of phytonutrient antioxidants.)

Food Pyramid Updates

Check for updates of the latest Food Pyramid. The *Food Guide Pyramid*, which was updated in April 2005 by the United States Department of Agriculture, is now called the *MyPyramid Food Guidance System*. Visit http://www. mypyramid.gov for updates of information.

About the Author

Anne Hart, popular full-time author of 64+ books and numerous magazine articles, is a member of the American Society of Authors and Journalists, the American Medical Writers Association, Mensa, and the International Documentary Association. She also holds a graduate degree and specializes in writing about nutrition, health, consumer behavior, and issues or controversies in the media.

Author's Web site: http://www.newswriting.net

Index

978-0-595-37823-4
0-595-37823-4

www.ingramcontent.com/pod-product-compliance
Lightning Source LLC
Chambersburg PA
CBHW030251290526
45785CB00001B/45